BREAK THE CHRONIC PAIN CYCLE

A 90-DAY PROGRAM
TO DIAGNOSE AND ELIMINATE THE ROOT CAUSE OF PAIN

SHEETAL DeCARIA, MD

MEGRINA PUBLISHING

PRAISE FOR
BREAK THE CHRONIC PAIN CYCLE

"This book should be read by every patient suffering from pain! Beyond breaking down the many reasons you are in pain, Dr. DeCaria provides easy-to-understand steps on how to eliminate it. A transformative guide to a pain-free life!"

—*JJ Virgin, 4x New York Times bestselling author, Celebrity Nutrition & Fitness Expert*

"Dr. DeCaria takes a root cause approach to managing chronic pain, from an integrative and functional medicine background. This book provides easy, effective, and natural strategies for those who want to heal their pain."

—*Amy Myers, MD, 2X New York Times bestselling author of The Autoimmune Solution and The Thyroid Solution*

"Chronic pain can be among the most debilitating and complex conditions in medicine. Dr. DeCaria's book *Break the Chronic Pain Cycle* touches on the many facets of pain including those that are structural, nutritional, and emotional. She does an excellent job relating how these causes can interplay and gives the reader practical steps to help them feel better safely."

—*Alan Christianson, NMD, New York Times bestselling author of titles including The Thyroid Reset Diet*

"A must-read guide for those suffering from chronic pain. *Break the Chronic Pain Cycle* is an evidence-based program that bridges the gap between conventional and functional medicine. This book is a blueprint to eliminate pain through easy-to-implement strategies that address the root cause of pain."

—*Madiha Saeed, MD, Bestselling author of The Holistic Rx*

"Beautifully written guide to conquering chronic pain and healing from the inside out. A must-read for anyone with pain!"

—*Ana-Maria Temple, MD, bestselling author of The Rule of 5: A Parent's Guide to Raising Healthy Kids in an Unhealthy World*

"As someone who has been dealing with chronic pain for several years, I am always looking for new books to help me feel good and eliminate pain. What I love about this book is the multi-pronged approach to healing that it teaches—combining the best of Eastern and Western medicine to provide an effective solution for anyone suffering from chronic pain. Western medicine has a tendency to compartmentalize pain—if your feet hurt, you see a podiatrist; if your belly hurts, you see a gastroenterologist; if you have recurring headaches, you go see a neurologist. It was so refreshing to read a book that approaches the concept of pain from a holistic perspective. It doesn't matter if your pain is in your foot, your arm, your hip, or your head. *Break the Pain Cycle* will help you get to the root cause of your pain and guide you through the steps you need to take to resolve it. Get ready to do some work—This book pushes you to reflect upon your current lifestyle and analyze the environment and conditions under which the pain began. Don't worry, you won't be overwhelmed at all. As you read each chapter, you will feel as if you have your own personal functional medicine doctor to guide you each step of the way in your healing."

—*Masumi Goldman, Bestselling author of Rise and Thrive*

"This book is a compendium of easily accessible and actionable tools for becoming pain free. Dr. DeCaria has created a 90-day program to help you regain your life. She describes the different pain syndromes and then provides clear solutions for you to implement immediately. I can't wait to recommend it to my patients!"

—*Jill R. Baron, MD, author of Don't Mess with Stress™—A Simple Guide to Managing Stress, Optimizing Health, and Making the World a Better Place*

HEALTH DISCLAIMER

Please consult your healthcare provider before making any healthcare decisions based on the information in this book and for guidance about a specific medical condition.

This book is intended to supplement, not replace, the advice of your healthcare provider. If you suspect a health issue, you should consult a licensed healthcare professional. The content in this book is provided as an informational resource only and is not to be used or relied upon for any diagnostic or treatment purposes. The information in this book does not create a patient–physician relationship and should not be used as a substitute for professional diagnosis and treatment. To protect patient privacy, all patient stories have been modified for all demographic factors (names, ages, etc.). Any resemblance, within this book, to real persons living or dead is purely coincidental apart from the story of the author. Brand and product names are trademarks or registered trademarks of their respective owners.

The author and publisher disclaim any liability, loss, or risk, personal or otherwise, that may be incurred as a consequence, either directly or indirectly, of the use and application of the contents of this book. The author has made every effort possible to research the validity of the information provided. The author and publisher assume no responsibility for errors, omissions, or inaccuracies contained in this publication. While this material is designed to offer accurate information at the time it was written, research in medicine is constantly evolving. Therefore, the reader must always check information provided with the most up-to-date published material and discuss any supplements or treatments with their physician. The author does not accept, and expressly disclaims, responsibility for any adverse effects or consequences resulting from the application of any advice, practices, or procedures described herein.

FREE GIFT!

If you would like to be emailed a free printable Companion Guide to use alongside this book, please visit https://www.drdecaria.com/breakthechronicpaincycle/ and fill out the contact form.

ACKNOWLEDGMENTS

I would first like to thank my family. To my beautiful daughters, who give me strength, joy, and laughter each day. To my parents, who worked tirelessly to give me a better life than they had. To my mother, for her kindness, love, endless support, and dedication. To my father, who showed me how rewarding this career could be and for supporting me through every stage of my life. To my big brother, for being an excellent role model and for always believing in me. And to my loving and devoted husband, who has stood by me and supported me as I pursued my dreams.

I also want to thank my mentors, teachers, colleagues, and friends for everything you have taught me throughout the years. As a physician, I am a forever student and eternally grateful to all of you for changing my life and shaping my practice.

And finally, I want to thank my patients, who provide me inspiration, motivation, and stories I will carry with me always. You are why I wrote this book.

TABLE OF CONTENTS

INTRODUCTION

"Natural forces within us are the true healers of disease."
—Hippocrates

After four years of college, four years of medical school, 16,000 hours of clinical training in anesthesia and pain management, and successfully passing three board exams by the American Board of Anesthesiology, I realized I only partially understood how to manage chronic pain.[1]

To put it in perspective, the FAA requires commercial pilots to train for 1,500 flight hours, which takes about two years, and pilots are extremely well trained in that time. Don't get me wrong. I did learn a lot in those 16,000 hours. Conventional medicine works incredibly well at treating acute pain, a predominant focus of my training. Opioids and procedures such as labor epidurals and nerve blocks succeed at virtually eliminating acute pain. But chronic pain is an entirely different ball game.

Chronic pain is an astronomical problem in the United States. Health economists have estimated the annual cost of chronic pain in the United States alone to be as high as $635 billion.[2] Technology has advanced tremendously, with new surgeries and procedures being developed each year, yet the number of people suffering from chronic pain continues to rise.

I was in college visiting my father's pain clinic when I first decided to go into pain management. Also an anesthesiologist and pain specialist, my father sat in a chair next to an elderly woman on a stretcher, holding one of her hands as he placed an intravenous catheter prior to her pain procedure. After he introduced me to her, she said, "Your father gave me my life back. And for that, I owe him mine."

Her statement continued to resonate with me as I went on to attend medical school and began my core rotations. I remembered her describing how debilitating arthritis pain had destroyed her life and how interventional procedures from my father allowed her to carry her grandchild for the first time. I remember hearing dozens of stories like that from my father and his patients. He had an unwavering enthusiasm and infinitely kind heart toward all his patients, traits I strive to mirror. He would often tell me, "Every patient has a story and a different reason for being in pain. My job is to listen to their story and find a way to help them."

Back then, I thought pain management would be that simple. I assumed that through procedures and techniques I would spend years mastering, all my patients would gain their lives back. I was naive, of course, but also optimistic and hopeful.

Since then I have learned that despite the billions of dollars spent trying to manage it, we have not conquered the problem of chronic pain for many of our patients. Western medicine does a great job of applying expensive Band-Aids (medications, surgeries, procedures) to help patients feel better in the short term. But then what? The Band-Aid falls off, and patients are back to suffering.

As I write this book, we are in the throes of an opioid epidemic. The 2018 National Incidence Drug Abuse Report states that 130 Americans die each day from opioids. In 2015, one out of every three Americans used prescription opioids.[3] As a consequence of the epidemic, and in an effort to mitigate overdoses and deaths, physicians are far more reluctant to write opioid prescriptions. Patients who had been prescribed opioids for non-cancer pain are now being told to find a way to self-manage their pain. They are lost and have no idea where to turn. Complicating their dilemma is the fact that the long-term use of opioids can actually trigger hyperalgesia or increased sensitivity to pain.[4] My approach provides a much-needed alternative.

As if we weren't already in trouble, the COVID-19 pandemic hit as I was working on this book. Its rapid spread has exposed large health disparity gaps amongst our communities. Reports are showing increasing opioid overdoses presumed secondary to rising rates of anxiety and depression, along with limited access to pain-relieving treatments. Studies predict that COVID-19 is going to leave our world suffering even higher levels of chronic pain than before, due to escalating levels of loneliness, isolation, physical inactivity, anxiety, and depression. Additionally, we are already seeing some patients develop a post-viral nerve pain syndrome following infection with COVID-19. Thus, now more than ever, we need to identify what is leading to chronic pain and provide a science-backed solution. With knowledge and tools come the ability to fight against these challenges and emerge pain-free.

Why is our country suffering an epidemic of chronic pain? I see three main reasons that we develop pain as a chronic disease and why we must look at it as more than just a symptom.

1. Our sedentary lifestyles and skyrocketing obesity rates adversely affect our posture and cause musculoskeletal imbalances. These predispose us to physical causes of pain.

2. Our overworked, high stress lives and emotional traumas result in chemical and hormonal imbalances linked to chronic pain.

3. Our diets and environmental toxins have led to continuous deep-rooted inflammation in our brains and other parts of our bodies, perpetuating a continuous pain cycle.

For these three reasons, the percentage of our population suffering from chronic pain continues to rise despite advances in modern medicine. Through my experience treating pain, I have identified three primary groups, or syndromes, that almost every chronic pain patient falls into. Many fall into more than one. Identifying your specific pain syndrome(s) is crucial to your recovery. My approach is based on getting to the root of the problem: removing and repairing the elements that have wreaked havoc over your body.

Many well-written books only address one aspect of pain treatment, such as physical exercises, mind-body therapies, or nutritional changes. But many patients need all of these, while others need only some. Far too often an author or practitioner, even if he or she claims to be "integrative" or "holistic," tends to have an underlying bias towards one discipline or another. This leads them to dismiss or ignore huge categories of possible therapies that may still be of benefit to you. How are you supposed to figure out which category you fall into? That is where this book stands apart. I am going to help you answer that question so that you can drive your care and finally get relief.

This book is an evidence-based resource from my experience as an integrative pain physician who has trained in both Eastern and Western medicine. I have also been a patient and navigated the system myself through my own journey with chronic pain.

This book is not a passive guide to healing or a quick fix approach. Relieving pain with an integrative, functional medicine approach requires effort on your part. This book will teach you to be a better patient so you can evaluate your own medical treatments, as well as provide self-management tools you can do on your own.

This book is divided into two parts. Part 1 will identify your main pain syndrome—the primary reason you are stuck in a chronic pain cycle. I will provide you with diagnostic tools to identify the cause of your pain and treatments and techniques you can implement to break your pain cycle. For many of you, you will see improvement after following these recommendations for forty-five days. For some, you may need to continue these treatments for three months to break your pain cycle.

Part 2 is a program designed to be followed for the next forty-five days that will further reduce your pain, as well as prevent future pain issues from developing. This section will teach you how to live well, use food as medicine, manage and minimize physical pain, lessen stress, and decrease toxin exposure. My hope is that after the ninety days, you will see substantial pain relief and choose to continue implementing your new lifestyle.

I am confident that this book will provide you with the tools you need to heal. I know you are reading this book because the system has failed either you or a loved one, and for that, I am truly sorry. It failed me as well.

But know that you are not alone, and your case is not hopeless. After reading this book, my hope is that you will be empowered with everything you need to self-manage your pain without reliance on medications or surgery. It will place you in the driver's seat of your own health. I am going to teach you to harness your body's own healing power through proven, scientifically-backed approaches. I will teach you how to lead a life of wellness, both to treat your current pain issues and prevent future ones. Preventative pain management is key to fighting the epidemic of chronic pain.

As Abraham Lincoln said, "The best way to predict your future is to create it." The person you are today will be entirely different than the person you will become once you break your pain cycle. I cannot wait to meet you on the other side.

PART 1

UNCOVERING THE ROOT CAUSE OF PAIN

CHAPTER 1

THE 21ˢᵀ CENTURY CHRONIC PAIN EPIDEMIC

"It is more important to know what sort of person has a disease than to know what sort of disease a person has."
—Hippocrates

A thirty-two-year-old female physician limped to her car after a grueling twelve-hour shift in the operating room. She had skipped lunch that day and had eaten some graham crackers and a soda from the doctor's lounge on the drive home. When she walked through the door, she had a rambunctious toddler waiting for her; and her next shift began. Motherhood. When her one-year-old finally dozed off for her nighttime slumber, the patient eased her swollen foot into a bowl full of ice water, hoping to numb the pain away. Exhausted, she slumped onto the couch. It was 8:00 p.m., and she no longer had the energy to exercise, knowing that her alarm was set for 5:30 a.m. Glancing in the mirror across the room, she saw the dark circles under her eyes and the stress lines on her face. Even though she knew she should take this time to meditate, she reached for the remote control and turned on Netflix.

It took me some time to step back and realize how many seemingly unrelated factors had contributed to this patient's pain. Because this time, the patient was me.

I vividly remember the day in October 2012 when my pain started. I was finally done with my training. All those years of agonizing over every exam score, accolade, scholarship, and award had led toward this one goal: to be a board-certified physician. I remember feeling relieved, but also like collapsing. I had spent my twenties studying, eating poorly, exercising occasionally, and being chronically stressed and sleep deprived. I had devoted every waking hour to my career and compromised my health and wellness along the way. I had little time to worry about what was happening to me when my focus was on my patients and medical education.

Not only that, but my personal life had crumbled as a result of my career. The list of significant life events I had missed was incredibly long: many of my baby's "firsts," friends' weddings, birthday dinners, and holiday celebrations, to name a few. I felt tremendous amounts of guilt that my training had led me to miss precious moments with my friends and family, and I was depressed and exhausted. By the fall of 2012, what should have been the happiest moment of my life with the successful completion of all my medical training, ended up being the lowest point of my life thus far. I didn't understand it at the time, but the culmination of all this emotional and physical distress had primed my body for entering into a chronic pain cycle.

The pain first started as a nagging ache in my foot after a Zumba class and a long day of carrying my toddler around. I had never truly experienced chronic pain in my life. Every issue I'd had in the past had, luckily, resolved itself quickly with no medications or medical attention. I had the usual severe back spasms from pushing heavy patient beds, a short bout of carpal tunnel during fellowship, and various other aches and pains, but they had all disappeared within a few weeks after doing the right exercises. I figured this would be the same, especially because there was no real "injury" involved. So I went about my life.

As the weeks went by, and I was working in an operating room day after day, I noticed the pain getting worse. Eventually, I could no longer walk without limping. I had to ice my foot to numb the pain so I could fall asleep.

After another few months of this pain, I decided it was time to see a foot specialist. I went to a highly regarded foot surgeon who took some X-rays and examined me for the ninety seconds allotted in our healthcare system. He told me my X-ray showed an old toe fracture and made a diagnosis without touching my foot. He instructed me to rest my foot by wearing a CAM (controlled ankle movement) boot for six weeks. He said I likely had sesamoiditis, or dancer's foot, which means inflammation of tendons near the big toe. There was no further instruction than that, no mention of the fact that hobbling on an uneven walk for the next six weeks would cause issues in my sacroiliac joint (a joint in my back).

I followed instructions and tried to be mindful of how I walked, despite his lack of instruction to do so, knowing the damage I was potentially causing. I made sure to use a shoe lift on my other shoe so I was walking evenly. The pain did not improve. In fact, it progressed to the point that my entire leg started to hurt. Over the next three years, I saw various specialists as my symptoms evolved to include hip and back pain. As if each represented an entirely separate problem, clinicians ordered MRIs of my foot, hip, and spine. Outside of some mild areas of inflammation, my MRIs looked okay. So I did more and more physical therapy, but the pain only worsened.

I saw multiple medical specialists at all the top hospitals in the Chicago area, and none of them had a treatment plan that gave me any relief. I also saw chiropractors, naturopaths, podiatrists, acupuncturists, physical therapists, massage therapists, myofascial release therapists, and holistic practitioners. Nothing worked. And with time, the underlying unidentified cause of my pain issues led to more and more pain.

Before I knew it, my symptoms had escalated even more. By the age of thirty-two, I suffered from heartburn, a very annoying twitch of my right eyelid, and chronic urticaria, or hives. I grew very frustrated with how difficult it was to navigate through the systems of complementary and conventional medical care. None of my providers talked to each other, and each one offered a different diagnosis.

If I was having such a hard time, how were patients expected to do it? Who was going to let them know that getting twenty-five treatments of spinal manipulation or acupuncture was not going to help them and might bankrupt them in the process?

While suffering from my own chronic pain, I dove into integrative medicine education, realizing how crucial it was that patients in pain find a provider who could guide them through this mess of a healthcare system. I learned ayurvedic approaches from practitioners who trained in India. I did a one-year faculty scholars program at Northwestern Osher Center for Integrative Medicine. I completed coursework through the Institute for Functional Medicine. I obtained certifications through the Academy of Integrative Pain Management and completed coursework through the American Academy of Anti-Aging Medicine. I read book after book, devouring as much knowledge as possible in a quest to find relief.

As I began to implement everything I learned, I realized the way conventional medicine approaches chronic pain was not working. Why? Because no one was addressing the root cause of pain.

HOW DID MY PAIN STORY END?

It took about four years. In that time, the providers I saw (both complementary and conventional) all came up with different diagnoses and treatment plans. Each focused on the symptoms. No one looked for the underlying cause. And guess what? None of the treatments worked. Many focused entirely on my foot, and then converted to focusing on my hip, and then my back. I spent thousands of dollars trying to find relief. But for those four years, I continued to suffer.

I was the first one to realize that the underlying causes were physical imbalances that started in my pelvis secondary to childbirth, as well as poor dietary habits leading to chronic inflammation and years of stress. Physical strengthening and mind–body techniques helped me get to about seventy percent relief. But the final approach that cured me was dietary changes. My case was relatively simple compared to those I see in my clinic, and even still, I needed to make a number of lifestyle changes to obtain relief.

It was not an easy road, and I still have relapses when I slack on my lifestyle choices and daily exercises. But the pain has never returned to a level that it impacts my life in any way. I am finally able to walk without a limp, I no longer wear a foot pad and ankle brace, I take frequent bike rides and hikes with my family, I no longer hobble out of work, I spend zero dollars on short term pain-relieving treatments, and as a nice side effect, my high cholesterol, eye twitch, hives, and heartburn have resolved. I now know what I need to do to avoid triggering my pain, and I healed myself without *any* of the medications, injections, or surgeries that were offered to me along the way.

Over the last thirteen years, I have successfully treated thousands of patients by blending Eastern and Western medicine. My conventional medical training rarely provided my patients complete relief, but once I developed this program, people began to heal.

Using a truly integrative approach is the only way to effectively eliminate pain long term. My goal is to share this program of wellness and healing with as many people as possible. I am writing the book I needed but could not find.

WHAT IS PAIN?

The International Association for the Study of Pain defines pain as follows: "An unpleasant sensory and emotional experience associated with actual or potential tissue damage, or described in terms of such damage."[1]

In most people, pain is temporary and a good thing. It is a way your body tells you something is wrong. When you break a bone or sprain your ankle, pain signals let you know to seek help and how to avoid worsening the injury. But for some people, the pain persists long after the initial injury has healed. You might wonder why. Why does your neighbor get a disc bulge and twelve months later is back to running a marathon, when you are crippled in pain with a "minor bulge," unable to leave your couch?

Chronic pain can wreak havoc on your mind and spirit. It can consume your entire being and become a vicious cycle you cannot escape. You become reliant on medication, even if it only relieves your pain partially or not at all. You start to fear moving or leaving your house since everything seems to exacerbate your pain. This isolation is also depressing and affects your social and family life, adding even more stress and anxiety. Those you love might worry about you, which can cause guilt and—you guessed it—more stress. Your sense of social isolation and alienation increases. You become more deconditioned due to lack of exercise, and more pain issues arise.

Traditional chronic pain management, which focuses on surgeries, procedures, and medications, will not heal this type of pain. This type of pain will require programs such as mine, with lifestyle and cognitive changes that go beyond the operating room and doctor's office.

Acute pain typically lasts shorter than three months and is often related to tissue damage that heals over time. Chronic pain is pain that persists beyond three to six months. Western medicine does an incredible job treating acute pain. Opioids are a vital part of what I administer during and after surgeries to instantaneously treat acute pain. Nerve blocks, where we inject numbing medicine around nerves, can completely numb a patient's body part so they can undergo a surgery wide awake with no pain whatsoever.

I experienced the marvels of modern medicine myself when I was in the final stage of labor (and in excruciating pain). In under ninety seconds, an epidural was placed, and the pain melted away. Modern medicine has incredible advancements for treating acute pain, but these same treatments do not effectively treat chronic pain.

OUR STATE OF HEALTHCARE

It seems that everyone in America either has pain, has had pain in the past, or will have pain in the future. In 2016, the CDC estimated fifty million U.S. adults suffered from chronic pain.[2]

The desire to treat symptoms through expensive quick fixes and to completely avoid investigating and treating the underlying cause has led to the issues our healthcare system faces today. Physicians feel an immense amount of pressure to make patients feel better immediately (following a ten- to fifteen-minute visit). And the quickest way to patient satisfaction is often masking the pain with a pill or attempting a quick-fix surgery or procedure.

The time it takes to uncover the root cause, the approach advocated in integrative and functional medicine, is not supported financially by our current insurance model. This is why most functional medicine and integrative practitioners, who spend thirty to sixty minutes with patients, rather than the five to ten minutes allowed under the insurance model, typically do not accept insurance. Many patients do not understand why this is, so I will take a moment to explain.

As time has gone on, insurance reimbursements for doctor visits have continued to decline, which forces doctors to see patients for shorter and shorter time intervals. This financial pressure is felt on an even larger scale by doctors who practice independent of a hospital system, because they are not able to negotiate to obtain more favorable contracts with insurance companies. For the same service, an independent doctor is often paid significantly less than one affiliated with a hospital or large group. This is why in 2020, many small medical practices are shutting their doors and joining larger corporations.

There are a large number of factors that affect why traditional doctors cannot sustain seeing patients for longer periods of time. For one, the average reimbursement of an annual well visit with your primary doctor is about $111. Most insurance payers will pay on average $140 for a forty-five to sixty-minute return visit and $75 for a ten- to fifteen-minute visit. When you factor in the cost of rent, staff salaries, equipment, electronic medical record systems, supplies, and medical school loan repayments, doctors simply cannot see a patient for thirty to sixty minutes with those types of reimbursements. Doctors in smaller practices are covering all their staff expenses on their own, with a nurse salary at approximately $62,000 per year (plus benefits) and the salary of an advanced practice nurse (NP) or physician assistant (PA) at approximately $115,000 per year (plus benefits), as well as the salaries of their medical assistants and receptionists.

Additionally, doctors face much higher costs to practice medicine than other healthcare providers. For example, a physician's malpractice insurance may cost $20,000–$45,000 a year (some higher-risk specialties like anesthesia and obstetrics can be even higher), while a physical therapist or acupuncturist may pay under $700 a year. That is quite a big difference and sheds light on why a physician needs to generate $300–$500 an hour instead of $100 an hour like most acupuncture sessions. There is also a big difference in the cost of medical supplies. A procedure needle, kit, and medications for a pain procedure may cost $40–$150, whereas acupuncture needles only cost a few pennies each.

With all the overhead costs mentioned above, physicians must see four to five patients an hour, at the minimum, to be able to even take home a profit over their expenses. If a doctor sees only one to two patients an hour, physicians accepting insurance would generate less income than their overhead and would quickly go out of business. This is why many doctors are either joining larger hospital systems, retiring early, or turning to concierge medicine and cash-only practices to provide more time with their patients.

It is important to also realize that a hospital bill is not the same as a physician bill. You may get a procedure or test at a hospital or surgery center and see an incredibly high bill of thousands of dollars. But most of that is the facility fee, or amount of the bill that goes in the pockets of the hospital itself and not directly to the physician.

For each full-time physician, studies show one and a half to two full-time staff members are needed simply to do the administrative tasks of prior authorizations and battling insurance companies. Because insurance reimbursements can be so complicated, many private doctors also use billing companies, adding to the overhead costs. I use an outside billing company that has two individuals specifically managing my account and one in-office staff member whose sole job is to sit on the phone battling insurance companies all day. Because she's doing this, she can't answer the phones, so I needed to hire someone else to do that. As you can imagine, costs add up quickly for a medical practice.

This does not even take into account the administrative tasks forced upon doctors that are unpaid. On average, a doctor will typically spend fifteen to twenty hours per week on top of their clinic time dealing with insurance company phone calls, documenting their electronic medical records, and making follow-up calls to patients and other doctors. This time is all unpaid and comes out of time they would otherwise spend doing something unrelated to work, like spending time with their children or participating in hobbies. As you probably know, many other professions charge by the hour (some by fifteen-minute increments), and very few do up to twenty hours of unpaid work per week.

Doctors also start out their careers with much higher levels of debt than most other professions. According to the Association of American Medical Colleges, the average medical school debt for the class of 2019 was $201,490!

As you can imagine, all this financial pressure does not leave doctors the option of spending more face-to-face time with their patients, even though that is what we want to do. It is why we chose a career in medicine—to help people!

Doctors are burning out at skyrocketing rates because they grow frustrated with the way our current healthcare system is dictating how we care for patients. The insurance model forces doctors to practice in a reactive way, treating illnesses and symptoms as they come up. Doctors simply do not have time to be proactive, teaching lifestyle changes to optimize health, because insurance companies don't pay for giving good advice. Consequently, a more proactive model with lifestyle counseling and prolonged visit times would force all independent doctors accepting insurance to go bankrupt and close their doors.

The sad reality is that doctors' suicide rate is amongst the highest of all professions, double that of the general population.[3] Unfortunately, doctors and patients are both suffering as a result of our current healthcare system.

HOW TO GET THE MOST OUT OF YOUR CONVENTIONAL HEALTH CARE VISITS

In an ideal world, everyone could see a functional or integrative medicine practitioner. Unfortunately, these cash-only practices remain financially out of reach for millions of patients who need them.

For those who cannot see a functional medicine or integrative practitioner, I recommend you do the following to try to get the most out of your conventional doctor appointments.

1. For each visit, pick one or two topics that are the most critical. Since the doctor only has five to fifteen minutes to see you, try to make the most of that visit.

2. Always come with a list of your current medications and supplements, including doses. Go through this list with your doctor, as some medications can cause joint pain, muscle pain, or headaches as side effects.

3. Come prepared with a pain diary of your symptoms, as well as all your records of prior treatments and medications. If you can create a document that shows all of this in a timeline fashion, it will save your doctor a lot of time and allow them to come up with a more effective plan. If you have had injections, be sure you know exactly what injection was done, when it was done, and if it worked for you. Have a list of what medications you have tried, how long you took each for, and whether it helped. Also make note of any side effects you

experienced. Many common medications can trigger joint, nerve, and muscle pain. Try to think back to when your pain started. If your pain started shortly after initiating a new medication, have a conversation with your doctor.

4. Come prepared with a list of your questions. Have the most important questions at the top of your list.

5. If you do not get through your list, schedule more frequent visits (either monthly or twice a month).

OPENING A NEW CHAPTER

Despite understanding the limitations within our conventional medical systems, I worked in conventional medicine for many years. Following my training at the University of Chicago for my anesthesia residency and at Northwestern University for my pain fellowship, I spent five years on faculty at the University of Chicago. During my time there, I did both anesthesia (putting patients to sleep for surgeries), as well as had my own pain clinic. I thoroughly enjoyed my time there, being surrounded by a highly academic and collegial group of colleagues. But I felt it was not the best practice structure for me. We worked at a fast pace, and although teaching trainees was an incredible gift, I missed the quality time I would spend with patients if I was in my own practice.

On top of that, I realized several years into my faculty position that there was a lack of integration between the complementary and conventional sides of medicine. This realization amplified as I journeyed through our healthcare system as a patient, and it led to me ultimately shifting my practice to a more holistic model.

All of this pushed me to do something doctors simply do not do anymore due to the increasing challenges of making this a sustainable business model. I opened up a solo independent practice: Revitalize Medical Center. As independent clinics around me were being swallowed up by powerful nearby hospital systems, I was going out on my own.

Despite extensive financial struggles from extremely high overhead and plummeting insurance payments, I began to see patients in my practice truly heal when they followed my lifestyle and dietary/nutritional recommendations. I decided to expand by offering additional programs, and people began to heal even more. Many stopped prescription medications they had been on for years and returned to activities they thought they would never be able to do again. I knew this was something I needed to share with patients beyond those I had the privilege to treat in person.

HOW TO USE THIS BOOK

You will begin by determining your pain syndrome(s). Based on that, you will read and follow the program outlined in your pain syndrome chapter(s). After you have determined what treatments you need to focus on based on Part I, you should implement these changes for forty-five days. After that period, you need to begin Part 2. Part 2 aims to repair and restore your body. These lifestyle changes need to be added to the treatments in Part 1 for another forty-five days to experience lasting improvement. It will take about three to four months to correct the abnormal physiologic patterns that have been established by your body and have resulted in this chronic pain disease state. Remember, reversing any chronic disease takes time. For some, it may take six months or longer.

I also want to make note that at the time of writing this book, I have no financial affiliations with any of the products, websites, or books I recommend. I am recommending them because I've researched and tested them and seen how they have helped my patients.

The internet is an incredible free resource with an abundance of information, but there is also a plethora of misinformation. When possible, I have tried to direct you to free, high-quality educational materials and videos to supplement this book.

My goal is to provide you with the tools you need to begin your journey to self-manage and heal chronic pain. This book will show you that the treatment course will not be a passive nor easy one. It will involve effort from you to make the necessary lifestyle changes, as well as effort to seek out the right practitioners who can offer effective treatments for your specific condition.

You are in control of your destiny. You are going to learn how to live again and how to cure your pain. When you see your doctors now, you will no longer take a passive role in your healthcare but will approach each appointment equipped with knowledge and confidence.

CHAPTER 2

IDENTIFY YOUR PAIN SYNDROME(S)

*"Healing is a matter of time.
But it is also a matter of opportunity."*
—Hippocrates

You are probably reading this book because you either fear the healthcare system, have tried things that failed, or had surgeries or procedures that have temporarily worked or, even worse, aggravated your pain further. You have all entered into the cycle of chronic pain, and no one has taught you how to break free of it.

Where you are on the chronic pain cycle spectrum will determine how well you will do with my system. If you are early on in the cycle, with pain symptoms that only partially interfere with your life, my system should leave you pain-free in three to six months. If you are further on in the cycle, with debilitating pain, even despite breaking the cycle, you may still be in some pain and require injections and/or medications. That is okay. Do not give up. This book can be used alongside other treatments.

I am going to begin this chapter with an assessment that sets your path for the remainder of the book. However, the assessment comes with a disclaimer. To truly find which category you fall into, you should be evaluated by a physician who is trained in identifying these issues. For those of you who do not have access to a functional or integrative pain physician, you should see a traditional pain physician and your primary doctor. The ideal starting point would be to see a board-certified pain specialist, a functional medicine practitioner, and a physical therapist. The three would need to work in tandem to identify the root cause of your symptoms.

For those suffering from pain related to cancer, fractures, acute pain, or infections, I urge you to seek conventional medical treatment, as this book is not aimed at those types of pain syndromes. However, if after appropriate treatment, you continue to suffer from pain, you may certainly benefit from the lifestyle changes taught in this book.

And as a physician, I must emphasize that the information contained in this book is designed to be used alongside care from a licensed professional. It was written with the goal that you can take an active role in your health, partner with your providers, and follow a proven pathway to healing. It was written to help all those suffering in chronic pain that are searching for answers and are constantly reaching dead ends. It is for those that may not even be suffering that much and have the attitude that they can "deal with it," but do not want to end up in the chronic pain states their loved ones are in. It is for those who want to know how to live better, feel better, and thrive without pain.

EVERYONE'S PAIN IS NOT THE SAME

Through my journey treating chronic pain, I have come to realize that there are three main syndromes that pain patients fall into: Physical Pain Syndrome, Mind-Body Pain Syndrome, and Central Pain Syndrome. Discovering which category a patient fits into can help ensure they are on the right path of treatment. Unfortunately, many practitioners are not trained at discerning which category a patient falls into. Traditional allopathic medical doctors tend to only look at the physical type of pain—because in our training, we learn that pain is your body's way of alarming us that something is wrong. We are taught that pain is physical and can be effectively treated with a pill or surgery. However, we are learning now that chronic pain is far more complex than that, involving a variety of other factors.

I have arrived at these syndromes through an approach that combines my conventional training with my integrative/functional medicine training. It is important to note that there is considerable overlap between the categories. Many patients fall into several of these categories but are only diagnosed with one. This leads to patients only treating one pain syndrome and ignoring the other, leading to limited relief.

Through my practice, I have found that over sixty percent of patients with chronic pain (i.e., pain that has persisted for over six months) fall into more than one of the following syndromes.

Before describing each pain syndrome, I'd like you to complete this exercise. This will allow you to evaluate your pain without any preconceived notions or premature self-diagnoses. For the first exercise, fill out the following.

Where in your body do you feel pain?

Knees, hips, collar bone, arms (mostly when holding my phone too long), shoulders

When did your pain start? What was happening in your life around this time?

started right after cruise with Mother

What does your pain feel like? Circle all of the words that describe your pain.

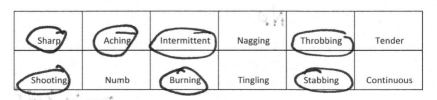

(Sharp)	(Aching)	(Intermittent)	Nagging	(Throbbing)	Tender
(Shooting)	Numb	(Burning)	Tingling	(Stabbing)	Continuous

What makes your pain better?

Walking (sometimes), prednisone

What makes your pain worse?

Movement, sitting still too long

Now that we have jogged your memory on the characteristics of your pain, let's proceed with the questionnaire to find your pain syndrome(s). There are three sections, which correspond to the three types of pain syndromes: Physical Pain Syndrome, Mind-Body Pain Syndrome, and Central Pain Syndrome. Circle the statements or questions that pertain to you.

1. PHYSICAL PAIN SYNDROME

a. Do you have burning/tingling/numbness that always follows a specific path either down your arm and/or leg or in your hands or feet? *Yes*

b. When you move a certain way, remain in a certain position, or use a specific part of your body, does it hurt (i.e., the same activity or activities always trigger your pain)? *Yes*

c. Has your pain been tied to a disorder or condition that you have (i.e., arthritis, ankylosing spondylitis, injury)? *Maybe*

d. If you or someone else pushes on a specific part of your body, does it hurt? *No*

e. Is there something on an imaging study (e.g., CT scan, MRI) that correlates to your pain (i.e., you have arthritis in your knee on an X-ray and pain in that knee when you walk)? *Don't know*

f.   When you take an anti-inflammatory medication such as Tylenol/Ibuprofen/steroid dose pack, does your pain improve?   *Yes*

g.   When you put ice or heat on the part of your body that hurts, does it feel better?   *Not sure*

2. MIND-BODY PAIN SYNDROME

a.   Was there a significant life event that took place in the weeks/days leading up to the onset of your symptoms? Example: divorce, death of a loved one, loss of job, sick parent or child, etc.   *Yes*

b.   Did you suffer any significant trauma as a child or adolescent? Example: physical or sexual abuse, death of parents, severe accident, etc.   *Yes*

c.   Is there a history of any of the following: frequent bouts of abdominal pain as a child, migraine headaches, irritable bowel syndrome, painful bladder syndrome, temporo-mandibular (TMJ) syndrome, or pelvic pain?

d.   Has no one been able to identify a physical cause for your pain thus far? Example: imaging studies like CT Scans, X-rays, or MRIs come back with fairly unremarkable or mild abnormal findings? Have doctors told you that there is nothing physical to explain your pain?   *Don't know*

e.   When you are feeling anxious or nervous, does your pain seem to worsen?   *Yes*

f.   Has your pain shifted in location over the years? Example: For part of your life, you had unexplained neck pain, and for another part of your life, you may have had unexplained back pain?   *No*

g.   Do you suffer from symptoms of anxiety and/or depression?

Yes

3. CENTRAL PAIN SYNDROME

a. Do you feel like you have pain all over your body or in many different unrelated areas? *Yes*

b. Have you been diagnosed with an autoimmune condition, fibromyalgia, migraine headaches, pelvic pain, or interstitial cystitis? *MCTD*

c. Are you hypersensitive to pain? Example: Something that should not cause pain, like someone pushing gently on your shoulder, causes you a lot of pain? *No*

d. Do you have discomfort in your bladder or pain when you urinate and/or do you suffer from irritable bowel syndrome, inflammatory bowel disorder, or have digestive issues such as constipation or diarrhea? *lately*

e. Do you have difficulty remembering things or feel fatigued/ exhausted all day long? *Sometimes*

f. Do you have swelling, changes in skin color/temperature, abnormal sweating, changes in hair or nails on an arm or leg? Did your pain start after an injury like a fracture or ankle sprain but has continued even after the injury healed? Did it start after surgery even after the wound healed? Have surgeries aimed at treating your pain failed?

g. Have conventional medical treatments like injections and medications failed to give you significant relief? *Yes*

If you answered "yes" to at least three questions within a category, you suffer from that pain syndrome. If you answered "yes" to even one or two questions, you likely will also benefit from treating yourself as if you were in that category. You may have early signs of that pain syndrome, which will only worsen if not treated.

BREAKING THE CYCLE

As stated earlier, the majority of patients in severe pain for many years fall into two, if not three, of these groups. However, early on in the pain cycle, patients may fall into just one category or syndrome.

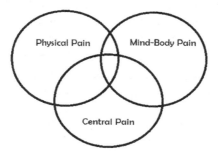

Figure 1. Pain Syndromes

It is important to note that if you fall into central pain, you likely also have some element of Mind-Body Syndrome.

Eventually, when pain has been around long enough (typically over three to five years), the circles in the diagram above tend to converge together, leading to an individual suffering from a pain cycle that involves all three syndromes.

WHAT TO DO NOW

Now that you know your pain type(s), you can navigate to the pertinent section in Part 1 and follow those treatment plans for forty-five days. If you fall into more than one syndrome, you can simultaneously treat each one. If after forty-five days, you are not beginning to see benefit, then I recommend you reach out to the providers recommended within your pain syndrome, as well as consider reading through the other syndromes, particularly the Mind–Body Syndrome, because many suffer from this unknowingly.

Then you will continue on to Part 2, which applies to everyone regardless of what pain syndrome they have. It begins with a twenty-one-day elimination diet that I strongly encourage everyone to do, regardless of the type of pain you have. However, if you choose not to, then please do the changes in the remainder of Part 2.

Part 2 of this book is useful for anyone, even those without pain, to learn to live healthier. If you are able to adopt a lifestyle filled with optimal nutrition, good sleep, stress management, and decreased external toxins and dietary inflammation, you are maximizing your chance to live a long and pain-free life. I encourage you to adopt these changes with your family members or close friends.

I hope this book teaches you the tools to self-manage pain, but my advice for those of you with severe pain is to start your treatment regimen with the help of the recommended professionals.

CHAPTER 3

PHYSICAL PAIN SYNDROME: UNDERSTANDING YOUR DIAGNOSIS

WRITTEN WITH REBECCA PAULIN-LISTON, PT, RYT

*"If your only tool is a hammer,
every problem looks like a nail."*
—Mark Twain

I met fifty-two-year-old Sylvia a few years ago. She worked in the environmental services department at the hospital. She had an incredible work ethic and told me that in twenty-five years, she had never called in sick until this pain started. By the time I met her, she had already been to the emergency room twice for her back pain. They had given her two rounds of heavy-duty oral steroids to slam her body into a state of anti-inflammation. This helped temporarily, but as soon as she stopped the steroids, the pain returned.

She had started physical therapy and had diligently completed three weeks of sessions. Unfortunately, her pain had worsened, and she had decided to take matters into her own hands and searched on Google to find a pain doctor. When she walked into my office, I immediately noticed her uneven walk. She sat down, dejected, and said, "I can't live like this." One doctor had told her she may need an exploratory hip surgery, and another had told her she may need a minimally invasive spine surgery. A third had said her imaging studies looked okay, and she just needed physical therapy. She didn't know what to believe.

We did a thorough history and physical exam and uncovered the source of her pain pretty quickly. Her pain was referred, so although she felt it in her hip, it was coming from her sacroiliac joint and a strained gluteus medius muscle. I did an injection that relieved her pain for several months. During that time, we worked on correcting her muscle imbalances through various strengthening and stretching exercises. After only one set of injections, exercise therapy, and a few extra tidbits found in my pain toolbox chapter (Chapter 17), her pain did not return.

SURGERY IS NOT ALWAYS A CURE

In some standard doctor's offices, the first person a patient is referred to when they complain of pain is a surgeon. However, in many cases surgery has been found to be ineffective and sometimes even more harmful than non-invasive treatments.

Did you know studies have been done on knee arthroscopies and shoulder surgeries and found no improvement when compared to patients that did not have any surgery?[1,2] A study called the FIMPACT trial looked at patients who received shoulder arthroscopies versus those who did not and found no difference.[3] That means those individuals had unnecessary surgeries, which is a big deal if we think about the time to recover from a surgery, the cost of a surgery, and the risks involved with surgery and anesthesia.

Not only are many surgeries unnecessary, but many diagnoses we find on imaging studies are also found to be incidental and not the actual source of pain. MRI studies have been done on professional baseball players with *no* shoulder pain and found forty percent had partial- or full-thickness rotator cuff tears in their dominant arm.[4] Despite these tears, these players have no pain and no limitations in moving their shoulders.

In 2007, the American College of Physicians Joint Clinical Practice Guidelines reported that, more often than not, back pain is not tied to a structural cause like a bulging disc. In one study, fifty-two percent of people with *no* low back pain were found to have at least one disc bulge.[5] In another study, looking at over three thousand patients with *no* symptoms of pain, they found disc bulge prevalence increased from thirty percent in twenty-year-olds to eighty-four percent for those eighty years of age. Disc protrusion prevalence increased from twenty-nine percent in twenty-year-olds to forty-three percent in eighty-year-olds.[6]

What does this mean? Many findings on MRIs are age-related changes and do not cause symptoms. So when those problems are treated through surgery, it doesn't fix the problem.

Every year, millions of people undergo these types of surgeries, yet only a small percentage of them actually need them. I see an alarming number of patients whose pain is not resolved with surgery, particularly those who have surgeries on their knees, shoulders, and spine. In these individuals, their pain is either unchanged by the surgery or relieved for a short period of time. This is because in these individuals we missed the underlying cause of what was actually causing their pain. I had a patient recently tell me the only time she was pain-free was the two hours after her spine surgery when she was heavily medicated from the anesthetic. After that wore off, her pain returned to the exact same level it was before the surgery.

Studies have repeatedly shown that back surgeries at long-term follow-ups of five to ten years do not show significant benefits over non-surgical management.[7] Knee arthroscopies have also been shown to provide only short-term benefit and no long-term benefit versus no surgery at all.[8]

I strongly believe that, with the exception of a medical emergency, every patient should see a physical therapist before undergoing these types of surgeries. I also believe that if your pain is severe enough to impact your life, you should see a board-certified pain doctor. It is a known fact among those of us who treat pain that the sooner we see a patient in physical pain, the greater success we have of treating it.

We should not be seeing you for the *first* time *after* you have a failed surgery. The earlier we see you, the less damage has been done, and the easier it is to break the pain cycle.

EXTINGUISHING THE ALARM, NOT THE FIRE

Imagine that you are asleep in bed when your fire alarm goes off. You jump out of bed and run into the room with the alarm. You notice smoke and smell burning, but when you call an expert and describe the horrible sound the alarm is making, they tell you to simply remove the batteries from the alarm and go back to bed. You do so and are immediately relieved from the annoying noise. If you shut the door, you can't even smell the smoke or feel the heat very much. You crawl into bed and go back to sleep. Likely, this story will not have a very happy ending. And although it seems a little ridiculous, it is often very similar to what is happening in regard to the standard treatment of chronic pain.

What I have found from treating thousands of patients is that the vast majority of patients are in physical pain due to muscular weaknesses or imbalances. These weaknesses and imbalances are rarely diagnosed and/or explained to patients by their doctors as the cause of their pain. Patients are rarely given exercise regimens, dietary recommendations, and lifestyle changes to eliminate their pain. Instead, they are given diagnoses and handed a prescription. And they are led to believe these diagnoses, such as a bulging disc, are the cause of their pain, rather than a symptom. Let's use an example to understand what I mean.

Let's say you have had back pain for many years. You see your medical doctor and he/she orders an MRI. Not surprisingly, the MRI comes back with scary words on it, and your chart now displays these "diagnoses": degenerative disc disease, herniated disc, and lumbar spinal stenosis. You have your label. With this label, you now get shuffled over to a spine surgeon, and fear develops based on this label. You are afraid to move a certain way, even afraid to sneeze because you may worsen your herniated disc. You stop exercising, and your pain worsens. You undergo back surgery, but six months later, you're back to suffering.

The issue is that you treated the symptom and not the cause. Your body, by developing this back pain and disc issue, has become engulfed in flames and is crying for help. But by having spine surgery, you were not extinguishing the source of the flame, which is a series of muscular imbalances in your body that led to the back pain in the first place. The result? With time, your body will again be engulfed in flames, and either the same or an adjacent disc will begin to have issues.

When the underlying imbalance persists, the pain either never goes away or returns in a short period (weeks to months) after surgery. If you're lucky, you may get five to ten years' worth of relief. But with no effort on your part, the pain will return in a much shorter time frame. The same disc or an adjacent one herniates (bulges out) and your pain cycle restarts. And as the imbalances persist, you may start to notice other issues down the chain, such as knee pain or foot pain. The same principles apply to surgeries to treat other areas of the body, such as knees, hips, and shoulders.

Here is a list of diagnoses commonly treated through surgery or pain medication, though in reality they are likely the result of physical muscular imbalances. You can see if you have been labeled with one of them.

- Carpal tunnel syndrome
- Radicular or sciatic pain
- Neck or low back pain
- Tennis elbow or golfer's elbow
- Plantar fasciitis
- Achilles tendonitis
- Shoulder or hip bursitis
- Tension or occipital headaches

Modern medicine has given us a quick surgery or pill for all of these—a temporary fix. Sadly, most of the time patients aren't even told that it is a temporary fix. This is likely because many doctors are not trained in diagnosing these imbalances, nor are they familiar with how to treat them. If you identify existing imbalances, you can repair current pain issues, and more importantly, prevent them from worsening.

Please note that the purpose of this chapter is not to say surgery never works. When a surgery is needed to correct something that is actually causing pain, then it is the right option. If a pinched nerve in your back is causing severe weakness in your leg, surgery may be needed to relieve that pressure and preserve your nerve so you can regain strength. However, if the surgery does not fix the underlying problem that led to the issue, it will not be a good long-term solution. You still need to address your imbalances even if you will have or have had surgery. I estimate that over half of patients with shoulder, knee, and spine issues that undergo surgery do not remain pain-free for longer than two to three years. This is because they had surgery to treat a symptom and not the underlying cause of their pain.

Before we dive into how to diagnose your physical pain condition, I want to make it clear that if you develop pain after an injury, you need to be evaluated first with an X-ray to make sure there are no broken bones. I also want to emphasize that if your pain occurs with any other red-flag symptoms—such as weakness of extremities, balance issues, impaired coordination, changes in bowel/bladder habits, fevers, concurrent unintentional weight loss, vision changes, rashes, nausea/vomiting, or numbness/tingling in the buttocks or perineum—you seek immediate attention by visiting the nearest emergency room. These are warning signs of possible dangerous health conditions that need to be addressed immediately. I have always said, for acute issues and acute pain, Western medicine not only works, but it is imperative and may save your life.

ANATOMY LESSON

Let's dive in. To understand physical pain, we need to do a very brief review of anatomy. This will help you understand the remainder of this chapter.

SKELETAL STRUCTURE

The adult human body has 206 bones. When two bones meet, it is called a *joint*. Joints often have a cavity with fluid in them and are divided into the following categories: fibrous, cartilaginous, and synovial. Ligaments are bands of connective tissue that connect to bones.

MUSCLES

Our body has over six hundred muscles. Muscles can be divided into subtypes: skeletal, cardiac, and smooth. Smooth muscles, such as your intestine or bladder, are controlled by our autonomic nervous system. Cardiac muscles are in our heart. Skeletal muscles attach to bones and ligaments and affect our posture, our strength, and how we move.

FASCIAL SYSTEM

Our fascia is a continuous sheath of connective tissue that passes through our bodies. The fascial system is crucial in causing pain and is often overlooked as a source of pain. Fascia has a higher number of sensory nerve endings than muscle and goes in tandem with muscular pain (hence the term *myofascial pain*).

NERVES

Nerves are bundles of fibers that send impulses of feeling to the brain or spinal cord and then send commands from there to muscles and organ systems.

WHO IS AFFECTED

Physical pain can affect us all—the stay-at-home mom who is constantly lifting her toddlers and doing housework all day, the athlete who is working some muscles and ignoring others, or the financial advisor spending hours a day hunched at a desk. We are *all* likely to face some level of physical pain in our lives, but for the majority of us, it is due to the posture we have when sitting and directly related to the amount of time spent in a sedentary state. Due to this, most of us are suffering from the same common muscular imbalances, which we will address in this chapter.

MUSCULAR IMBALANCES

What I have seen is the majority of patients have two main issues: (1) tight neck and shoulder muscles from being hunched over and (2) rotated, tilted, or uneven pelvic rims due to weak gluteal, pelvic floor, and leg muscles. Both of these issues lead to muscular imbalances, which lead to pain. The upper body imbalances lead to headaches, neck pain, arm pain, and mid-back pain. The pelvic and gluteal imbalances lead to low back pain, hip pain, knee, and foot pain. Chronically tight and/or weak muscles lead to dysfunctional movement patterns that eventually lead to structural damage in discs, joints, muscles, and bones throughout the body.

I am going to teach you how to identify and treat some of these common issues.

THE PHYSICAL EXAM: FINDING THE "PAIN GENERATOR"

The first step of my algorithm for physical pain is to look for a "pain generator." A pain generator is a part of the body that is causing physical pain. I begin by asking specific questions and gathering a patient's history. The second, equally important step is a physical exam. The pain generator refers to the part of your body causing the pain. It may be a symptom of another underlying issue tied to an imbalance in another part of your body, or it may be the sole cause of your pain. The pain generator can sometimes be identified by an imaging study, but believe it or not, many times findings on an MRI or X-ray do not correlate with one's pain. Due to this, you cannot make diagnoses based on an imaging study alone. I prefer the method of using a combination of the history, physical exam, and injections to find the pain generator. This chapter will teach you how to do this yourself.

An important point to note as you read this chapter is that often people have multiple pain generators. These "hot spots" can be fairly predictable and indicative of specific imbalances, which can often be due to one underlying root cause even though the pain presents in different areas. Think of your body as a kinetic chain of dominos. Each area of pain is a separate domino, whether it be your spine, your hip joint, your knee joint, etc. And although they appear as separate areas, they are actually connected and impact one another. All it takes is one domino to get unstable and fall over to then knock down the rest of the dominos.

Unfortunately, in the design of our current healthcare system, patients are told, "Oh, you have hip bursitis, arthritis in your back, and tendonitis in your foot. You need to see three separate specialists." When in fact, all of these are tied to one another. For example, weak gluteal muscles and an uneven pelvis could lead to all of these issues. However, when looked at as entirely separate entities by three different specialists, the root cause will be missed. In other words, the source of the "flame" will persist despite temporarily extinguishing each mini fire.

INJECTIONS: CONFIRMING THE "PAIN GENERATOR"

If you have been suffering from chronic pain for some time, you have likely received an injection or two. In my clinic, I use injections to target what I believe from my history and physical exam to be the pain generator. The injections, depending on what is injected, work in different ways. A steroid can be administered to decrease inflammation, or a substance such as platelet-rich plasma can be injected to try to regenerate tissue.

Even more commonly, injections contain local anesthetic, or numbing medicine, such as lidocaine. The numbing medicine is what physicians often use to identify the pain generator because it works right away. This pain generator could be a muscle, a disc in your spine, a joint, a nerve, or something else. Following my injections, patients wait a short period, and then I ask them to do pain-provoking maneuvers and see if they feel better. We also give them a pain diary to fill out so they can assess how much better they feel and what still hurts, if anything.

This approach is very important in helping to identify and treat pain effectively because almost every injection includes numbing medicine, and if the area injected is the pain generator, the pain should disappear within five to ten minutes of the injection. This relief should last for a predictable length of time based on what anesthetic was used. (For example, lidocaine should give relief for one to two hours.) If injecting the area you suspect is the pain generator does not provide relief, it does not matter what your MRI or X-ray shows, the pain is not coming from that area. This approach should help to avoid unnecessary surgeries.

You can see that identifying the pain generator is a vital part in identifying the underlying cause of pain. Once you identify the pain generator(s), either by physical exam or an injection, you can use the tools described in this chapter to find out what imbalances led to those areas of pain and treat them accordingly.

George was a patient who came to my clinic too late. He had fallen down at work and started having back pain. An MRI showed a small disc protrusion at the L5-S1 level (the bottom of the spine). A doctor had performed an epidural injection at that level that had not provided relief. So George had surgery. Unfortunately, he woke up and he said the next day he noticed the pain felt the same as before the surgery. When he came to see me, I asked him if the epidural had provided *any* relief, even for two hours. He said no. He also told me that no one had asked him that. They had just asked him if it worked, and when he said no, he was scheduled for surgery. This is unfortunate because, from the fact that the injection had provided no relief even during the first two hours when the numbing medicine was working, I knew then that his pain was not coming from his spine. We did an exam, and it clearly showed his sacroiliac joint was the source, a joint that joins the pelvic bone to the lower part of your spine. It was a shame he underwent an unnecessary surgery, because the fusion surgery he had was actually going to worsen his sacroiliac joint pain over time.

Here are examples of procedures that can be used to identify pain generators. This is not a comprehensive list, as there are over 180 injections that can be done to treat pain. I am going to list the most common injections done and ones that have been used successfully to diagnose pain generators.

HEAD/NECK:

- Occipital nerve block
- Supraorbital nerve block
- Trigger point injections
- Botox injections for migraines
- Cervical spine injections (targeting various parts of the spine)

ARM:

- Carpal tunnel injection
- Lateral/medial epicondylitis (tennis/golfer's elbow)
- Cubital tunnel injection
- Shoulder Injection (variety of joints and ligaments of shoulder)
- Trigger finger injection
- Stellate ganglion block for CRPS/RSD of arm

CHEST WALL PAIN:

- Sternoclavicular joint injection
- Intercostal nerve blocks (rib pain)

ABDOMEN:

- TAP blocks for abdominal wall pain or post-abdominal surgery pain
- Celiac plexus for pancreatic cancer/masses/abdominal pain
- Superior hypogastric for various cancers in lower abdomen
- Ilioinguinal/iliohypogastric/genitofemoral nerve blocks

LOW BACK/BUTTOCK PAIN:

- Lumbar spine injections (variety can be done to target discs, nerves, joints)
- Ganglion impar for cancers
- Coccyx injection for tailbone pain

HIP/PELVIS:

- Hip joint injection
- Saphenous nerve for pain on inside of thigh
- Trochanteric bursa for pain on outside of thigh
- Piriformis muscle injection for buttock pain
- Pudendal nerve block for pelvic pain
- Sacroiliac joint injection for hip/groin pain

LEGS:

- Lumbar sympathetic block for CRPS/RSD
- Knee injections
- Lateral femoral cutaneous nerve for nerve compression at waist by belts, etc.

FEET:

- Achilles tendon injection
- Plantar fasciitis injection
- Toe joint injections
- Anterior and posterior tarsal tunnel injections
- Sesamoiditis (dancer's foot) injection

Once an injection is done and the pain generator identified, you can work closely with a physical therapist on exactly what exercises to do to correct what led to that issue.

DO INJECTIONS FIX MY PAIN?

Injections are typically Band-Aids over your pain symptoms. They will make you feel better, but they are not curing the underlying issue. If your doctor successfully identifies your pain generator and injects this area, you should obtain relief for physical forms of pain for variable lengths of time. At the very least, if the pain generator is treated, you should obtain relief for the duration of the numbing medicine. This relief typically lasts two to six hours. It is the long-term relief that is variable. If it is an inflammatory issue, you will obtain relief if a steroid was injected. This relief will last for approximately one to four months due to the anti-inflammatory effect. If we do an ablation of nerves that control sensation—a process that involves a heated tip needle to create a lesion—patients get relief until the nerves regrow (six to twelve months).

The goal with getting injections and procedures is to provide a diagnosis and make you feel better. But the real goal is that, while you are feeling better, you use that time to target and correct the underlying issue so the pain does not return once the injection wears off. If you simply get an injection and make no other changes, your pain will return.

YOUR INJECTIONS WERE WORKING AND NOW THEY'RE NOT

"Doctor, my injections were initially working well. I would get six months of relief. Now I only get a week, max. Why?"

I get asked this question *all* the time in my clinic. There are multiple reasons, and a doctor can help tell you which pertains to you. For some, your muscle imbalances and/or poor posture, when uncorrected, continue to progress over time. Depending on what muscles are involved, these imbalances can even lead to conditions such as herniated discs, compressed nerves, premature joint degeneration, and chronic headaches. The longer these imbalances go untreated, the worse they get, and the more likely you are to develop a new pain generator (now your back *and* knee hurt). When this occurs, relief from your injections will last for shorter periods.

Another reason is that some areas begin as inflamed, but even when that inflammation subsides, the pain persists. This is typically a result of the pain cycle progressing to involve components of Mind-Body Syndrome and Central Pain Syndrome (future chapters).

For those who have had surgery, the pain may be caused by scar tissue compressing on a nerve. This type of pain is very difficult to treat because it typically will no longer respond to steroids, and additional surgery only causes more scar tissue.

For some, the prognosis is a bit grim. Obesity combined with muscular imbalances has led to a rapid rise of degenerative osteoarthritis. This "wear and tear" arthritis primarily affects knees and hip joints. If you have advanced arthritis, you may have been told your joints are "bone on bone." For these folks, injections stop working as the joint space gets smaller and smaller. There is no longer any inflammation there, and you are injecting steroids for no reason. For some of these patients, there are other options beyond steroid injections that can still provide some relief. Doctors can inject synthetic gels to mimic joint space fluid or perform an ablation, where we burn nerves that provide sensation to a joint. But while these longer-lasting procedures are giving you six to twelve months of relief, your joint is continuing to degenerate unless you have corrected your imbalances and lost weight. As a result, eventually, these stop working as well, and you will need a joint replacement. But remember: if the underlying issues remain the same, your joint replacement could fail as well!

THE PHYSICAL EXAM

I cannot state enough how important the physical exam is to making a diagnosis. Unfortunately, in our conventional system, the majority of pain diagnoses are made based on MRI and X-ray reports alone. Many patients will have seen several doctors and no one has done a thorough physical exam. Without a physical exam, including palpation, or applying pressure, to the affected area, as well as specific tests, there is no way to make a diagnosis with certainty. As stated above, injections can be done to aid in the diagnosis, but even injections do not diagnose the root cause of *why* an area is causing pain. You must do an exam.

MUSCLE IMBALANCES

Before we dive into how to do the exam, we need to understand what we are looking for: muscle imbalances.

We spend so much of our lives hunched over our desks, sitting with bad posture, and suffering from skyrocketing rates of obesity. In these positions and conditions, some muscles get overly tight, and others overly stretched. On top of this, our joints are facing extreme pressure due to the excess weight. This extreme pressure on top of existing muscle weaknesses causes immense stress on our bodies. The result of these imbalances are numerous pain syndromes.

THE KEY TO FINDING RELIEF IS REGAINING BALANCE

It is important to think about your body as a collection of muscles that balance each other out. There are groupings of muscles: the muscles on the front of your body must balance those of the back of your body, and muscles on the left side should balance those of the right side. When there is an imbalance, one muscle group gets shorter and the other gets longer, or one gets stronger and the other weaker.

If you look at yourself slouched in the mirror from the side view, you will notice your chest is sunken in (i.e., the chest wall muscles are in an overly shortened position), and your back, neck, and shoulder muscles are elongated and stretched out. In this position, your chest wall muscles are in a shortened position and not being used properly, and your back, shoulder, and neck muscles are being used incorrectly. The goal is for your muscles to remain in a neutral, or resting, position most of the day.

You might be wondering, why then do my "stretched out" muscles feel so tight? The issue is that when muscles are stretched, they lose oxygen supply (ischemia), and when this ischemia takes place, the muscle tightens and causes pain. In my experience, this condition—myofascial pain syndrome—is the cause for the majority of chronic pain, particularly chronic neck and back pain.

Why is it that doctors gloss over muscle pain? Why is it that this seems so obvious and should be easy to treat, but doctors will rarely tell you that it is your diagnosis? A lot of conventional medical doctors do not believe that muscles can be the origin of severe pain, and many do not believe muscles can spasm over nerves and cause neuropathy or nerve-like pain as well. I believe they can, and do, at a higher frequency than is diagnosed. If we discovered these issues more frequently, we would treat pain more effectively and avoid unnecessary surgeries.

Unfortunately, muscle pain syndromes are quite challenging to study and poorly understood. Studies have shown decreased oxygen flow to muscle cells in patients with back pain.[9] Other studies have found local degenerative changes and swelling of muscle fibers in patients with back pain. In the more chronic stages, fibrosis, or scarring, develops in the muscle.[10]

Muscle pain is difficult to treat with Western medicine approaches because they rely predominantly upon costly tools such as MRIs or X-rays to make a diagnosis (rather than using a hands-on physical exam). MRIs and X-rays are not able to show muscle pain as a diagnosis. Then based on the results of these imaging studies, Western doctors rely on medications and surgeries for a solution. We've already discussed the drawbacks and risks of unnecessary surgeries.

Furthermore, many common medicines used for muscle pain are not very effective. For example, medications touted as muscle relaxants do not always work well. They work centrally on your brain, rather than relaxing your muscles directly. A true muscle relaxant would relax all your muscles, including those that enable you to breathe. True muscle relaxants are used by anesthesiologists in the operating room when we are performing surgeries. Another factor discouraging muscle pain as a diagnosis is that the medical system makes more money from costly surgeries than from time spent teaching focused exercises and encouraging lifestyle changes.

Determining the correct and precise area of muscle pain rather than erroneously identifying a structural issue, such as a bulging disc or arthritic joint, as the cause of pain is immensely important, not only to successfully treat pain, but also to prevent an unnecessary surgery that could cause more pain.

I am going to teach you simple tools to check if your pain is originating from muscles and not a structural issue like a herniated disc or arthritic joint. There are a handful of syndromes that are often misdiagnosed as the cause of one's pain, leading to millions of unnecessary surgeries. They include misdiagnoses like a torn meniscus, rotator cuff tear, arthritic "bone on bone" joints, and herniated discs. We are going to look at these commonly misdiagnosed syndromes one by one, teach you physical exam tests to make that distinction, and provide you with exercises to correct your imbalances.

The aim of the next chapter is not to go over every single Physical Pain Syndrome. The goal is to go over the physical conditions that are often misdiagnosed, to teach you how to identify your imbalances, and to give you exercises to correct them so you can treat the root cause of your pain. This approach will not only treat your current pain issue, but prevent future pain issues.

COMMITMENT

It is important to remember that to truly heal physical pain, you will need to invest time every day to doing the recommended stretches and every other day to doing the corrective and maintenance exercises. These must be done for months because our bodies will automatically revert to our imbalances due to muscle memory from years of poor posture and patterns of use and disuse. On top of that, our modern, digitized worlds continuously place us in these positions, so even after we correct them, we will constantly retrigger imbalances. The only way to correct them is to reset and rebalance regularly. The commitment is about fifteen to twenty minutes a day, so I hope you are willing to stick with it. Once your imbalances are corrected, Chapter 13 provides a daily exercise/strengthening program you should implement to prevent future physical pain issues.

CASE STUDY

A sweet couple in their eighties came to visit me in my clinic. As they sat in the waiting room, they both struggled to fill out their pain history questionnaire. Thirty minutes passed, and their paperwork remained blank. I asked my staff to assist them. My medical assistant reported that the couple told her they had no pain. I invited them to the exam room, curious to learn more about their story. They sat in front of me, holding X-ray reports that stated they both had severe degenerative arthritis. A surgeon had already scheduled their knee replacements, but they came in for another opinion.

I asked them about their pain, and they reported they had no pain. I asked them about what physical activity limitations they had, and they reported no pain with walking or stairs. They did say they had steroid injections into their knees that didn't seem to change anything, since they had no pain before the injections. I inquired as to why they even had the knee X-rays, and they said at one point the wife had mild pain that lasted a few months, during which time she did some physical therapy and had the X-rays. However, the pain resolved with muscle strengthening. The husband reported his doctor had X-rays done as part of his routine exam after he saw his wife had such severe arthritis. They reported their knee arthritis did not limit their activities, and they still walked about a mile each day without pain. Their physical exam showed some mild limitation at the extremes of their knee range of motion, but this did not elicit pain. I told them, "Please do not have surgery. Go live your life, continue your daily walking, and stay in good health, away from an operating room."

Stories like this display what is wrong with our system. People are treating images and not patients. I hope as we dive through the next chapter, we save you from an unnecessary surgery (or direct you to one that will provide long-term relief).

CHAPTER 4

PHYSICAL PAIN SYNDROME: CORRECT YOUR IMBALANCES

WRITTEN WITH REBECCA PAULIN-LISTON, PT, RYT

*"The pain you feel today is
the strength you'll feel tomorrow."*
—Anonymous

TAKE YOUR OWN SYMPTOM HISTORY

Let's start by taking a history. Think about what is affecting your symptoms. Do certain activities make your symptoms better or worse? Does massage help temporarily? Is your pain worse after resting or sleeping when the muscles aren't being used but improves fifteen minutes or so after you are up and moving? Does sitting in a sauna help? You can refer back to your notes from Chapter 2.

Why does your pain feel worse in the morning? Your muscles are not getting blood flow overnight, so they shorten and contract, leading to pain until you get moving again. Does your pain improve with a massage, heating pad, or hot shower? These are all indications that your pain is coming from muscles, as heat provides improved blood flow, and a massage can release areas of muscle tension.

INSTRUCTIONAL MATERIALS

All of the exercises I reference in this chapter can be found in the Exercise Appendix. The exercises are numbered (E-1, E-2, etc.) and will be referenced throughout the chapter. Also, videos demonstrating many of the exercises can be found at www.drdecaria.com/exercises/.

CORE OF YOUR FUNCTIONAL EXAM

Since many of us have the same imbalances, the core of the functional exam is the same for everyone. After you do the core exam, you can skip to the section with your specific pain symptom for more instructions.

1. GAIT ANALYSIS

The first thing to do is look at how you are walking (gait). Your gait can tell a lot about the underlying cause of your pain symptoms. Ideally, you have someone (or set your phone to do this) take a video of you walking with fitted clothing or shorts and a tank top. Try to focus your attention on the hips down to the feet. Take the video from the front and back views and see if you notice that one or both feet turn inward or outward. Take note if one side of your pelvis or hip appears higher than the other. Take note if you are limping. These can all be indicators of muscular imbalances. Take a video with and without shoes. See if your feet appear to be in equal position and have equal arches. Have your partner check if your feet are flat and have lost the arches. Notice these findings and compare them to how things look in the following tests.

2. POSTURAL ANALYSIS

For good posture, the muscles on the front of your body should balance and be equal in strength to the muscles in the back of your body (see Figure 2 versus Figure 3).

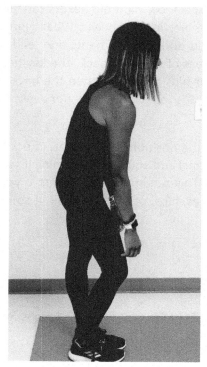

Figure 2. Poor Posture

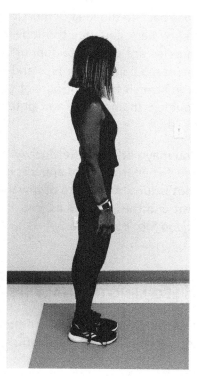

Figure 3. Good Posture

Our lifestyles lead to an altered forward shoulder posture where the chest, shoulder, and biceps muscles are stronger than our shoulder blade and triceps muscles. The way to correct your posture is to regain this balance and return your muscles to neutral. Even if you do not have pain in your neck and shoulders, but you notice you are hunched forward, I suggest you do the *scapular squeeze* (E-2).

For some, the entire pelvis is rotated forward. This can be seen in individuals with an excessive lumbar curvature of the spine (your stomach appears to be pushed out). How does this happen?

We spend a lot of our day sitting. In this position, your quadriceps, hip flexors, and low back muscles are tight and contracted, and your gluteal and hamstring muscles are stretched and not being used. This goes back to the idea of muscle imbalance. Tight hip flexors can lead to low back pain due to mobility issues in your pelvis. Weak gluteal muscles are unable to support you during movements and lead to increased pain in your hips and areas of your low back. The key here is to stretch the front part of your hips and strengthen the back of your legs (hamstrings) and gluteal muscles. Do the *posterior pelvic tilt* (E-24).

You may notice a difference with the position of your feet. Check to see if your arch height appears normal and equal, and examine if your foot is turned outward or inward. This can impact symptoms in your feet and toes, as well as your knees, hips, pelvis, and back. If so, do *tripod foot posture* (E-29).

3. LEG LENGTH ANALYSIS

Next, it is important to see if there is an issue at your pelvis causing a discrepancy in your leg length.

Lie flat on your back and have someone else place their thumbs on the pointy bones on the inside of your ankles. These are the malleoli. Have them bring your feet together and see if their thumbs are perfectly lined up. If they are not, see which thumb is either too high or too low, and that will tell you which side is shorter. This same issue can also be diagnosed with the posture analysis if you see one hip hiked up higher than the other.

Although it is possible that you have a leg length discrepancy from birth, the majority of the time, I see patients who have issues due to a muscular imbalance of their quadratus lumborum muscle or psoas muscle.

Although it can help in the short term, a lift in one shoe is a Band-Aid over the symptom. Stretching the muscles is actually what is needed to bring the balance back.

If you have a leg length issue, please do the following stretches (E-23 *quadratus stretch*, E-13 *child's pose*, and E-21 *psoas stretch*). Notice which side feels tighter and does not move as far, and spend more time stretching that side.

These types of issues can present as sacroiliac joint pain, back pain, hip pain, and even foot pain. See below for further exercises for your specific condition.

4. PELVIC ROTATION ANALYSIS

Stand up straight. Place your hands on the two bony protrusions in your back, right above your pelvis—they feel like two peas under your skin on the left and right. These are your posterior superior iliac spines (Figure 4). See if they are sticking out the same amount. See video: *Assessing Hip and Pelvis.*

If one side seems less pointy or deeper in the tissue, there is possibly an anterior (frontward) or posterior (backward) tilt or shifting of your pelvis leading to imbalances.

You should also feel the bony rim at the front of your waist to see if your hands are even with one another (Figure 5). If the two sides do not match, you likely have some form of pelvic rotation.

Another test to check if you have a rotated pelvis is to lie on your back and see if one leg rotates out farther than the other. If they look uneven, this can happen from your lower leg or from your pelvis. Take a look at your knee—is it pointing up to the ceiling but your foot has rolled out? This means the rotation is coming from your lower leg and is most likely due to the way your lower leg has formed. This is less common and more difficult to treat, so we won't address that here, but it can be addressed with a physical therapist. Most of the time, the asymmetry is due to a pelvic rotation, and one leg will be rotated out farther than the other leg.

For many people, pelvic rotation is an acquired condition. It can happen during or after childbirth when women's pelvises are prone to injuries. It can happen as a result of trauma. For others, it is a result of poor posture for many years. I have found it to be extremely common.

Often the pelvis can be in rotation due to imbalances in the muscles attaching to the hip and pelvis. Exercise: *piriformis stretch* (E-22) and *glute activator* (E-25).

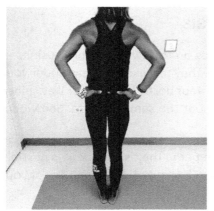 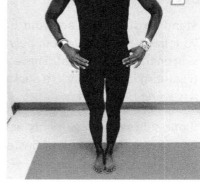

Figure 4. Feel Posterior Pelvic Rim   **Figure 5. Feel Anterior Pelvic Rim**

5. PELVIC TILT ANALYSIS

This is a very common finding I see in terms of pelvic issues.

The pelvis can tilt forward (anterior) or back (posterior). If it tilts forward, then you have an exaggerated curve of your lower back. When this happens, it is because the psoas muscle and hip flexor muscles are stronger and tighter than your gluteal and buttock muscles.

If you have an anterior curve, do these exercises: *posterior pelvic tilt* (E-24), *psoas stretch* (E-21).

If you have a posterior pelvic tilt, it may appear that you have a flat lower back. When this happens, it is because the hip flexors lengthen too much and your gluteal muscles are more contracted.

If you have a posterior curve (a flatter lower back), do these exercises: *knee to chest stretch* (E-16), *cat/cow pose* (E-5).

6. PALPATION AND STRENGTH

Palpation refers to pushing on an area to see if it is sore.

Strength testing refers to checking how strong a muscle group is. This is graded from no movement to being able to move it with someone else holding resistance against that muscle. I will not go over how to grade it, but the simple idea is if you cannot hold strength in a muscle with someone holding resistance against your motion, you have some form of weakness. A partner can check if one side is stronger than another. Another important thing to keep in mind when doing strength testing is that you should try to hold, even if it is painful, in order to assess true weakness.

7. RANGE OF MOTION ANALYSIS

The *range of motion* (ROM) test will aid in distinguishing genuine structural issues from muscle weakness or imbalances. ROM is broken down into active and passive range of motion. For the purpose of this chapter, this test is specific for a joint (such as your knee, hip, shoulder). A joint has a normal range of motion, but each person has different "normal" ranges.

A good way to test is to compare the affected or painful side with the non-painful side so you can see what your normal range of motion is. Active range of motion is the range of motion your joint has when you are moving it yourself. Passive range of motion refers to someone else moving your leg from full flexion (bent) to full extension (joint fully straight) and seeing how far they can move it. You want to compare active and passive ROM for both right and left joints. For true structural issues in a joint, active and passive ROM will produce the same results, and both of these tests will show reduced range of motion. However, if the active ROM is decreased but the passive ROM is full or the same as the non-painful side, the issue is more likely related to muscles around the joint (i.e., you need physical therapy, not surgery). For clarity on the full range of motions of each joint, check out the following videos: *Shoulder Joint Movement* and *Hip Joint Movement*.

COMMONLY MISDIAGNOSED SYNDROMES THAT CAUSE PAIN AND EXERCISES TO TREAT THEM

My general rule of thumb with anything physical in my program, whether it is a stretch or an exercise, is this: If it hurts, don't do it. Stop and consult a professional. I have seen plenty of injuries from improper exercise techniques or overstretching. Also, if you do not exercise regularly, start with the assistance of a physical therapist. I personally feel everyone should have an evaluation by a physical therapist at the first sign of pain symptoms.

Let's dive into the commonly misdiagnosed syndromes from head to toe. This list is certainly not comprehensive for every possible physical ailment. That would require its own book(s). However, I chose to cover the diagnoses that I feel are most commonly seen and also often misdiagnosed as structural when they are in fact muscular. By uncovering the root cause of these issues, we can eliminate these persistent pain syndromes, while avoiding a significant number of unnecessary surgeries and medications.

HEADACHE/NECK PAIN: CERVICAL SPINE OR MUSCULAR ISSUE?

PHYSICAL EXAM

First, look in the mirror and do a postural analysis. Are your shoulders even, or is one higher than the other? If they are uneven or your head at rest is tilted to one side, your issue may be a short scalene and levator scapulae. That is your muscle imbalance. This can present as neck pain, chest pain, or shoulder pain. It can also cause tension, migraine, or occipital headaches.

Do you have pain on one side or both sides? If it is on both sides, it is likely related to poor posture causing muscular imbalances from hunching forward all day. If it is on one side, it may be due to the way you sleep or your position during certain activities. This is a right/left imbalance. It is important to keep in mind that pain from muscular issues can also cause decreased spinal range of motion. Your neck may not move as easily if the muscles are very tight.

Often, the levator scapulae and trapezius muscles are the source of muscle pain. The suprascapular nerve can even become trapped in your shoulder blade muscles and cause tingling and pain that can be erroneously attributed to a pinched nerve in your neck.

Next, I will walk you through the specifics of the physical exam.

1. **Photo.** Take a side photo of your posture and see if your shoulders are hunched over or if your head is learning forward (ear forward compared to your shoulder).

2. **Palpation.** Feel for any areas of tension. If you feel knots or any areas that reproduce your pain by pushing on them, you likely have muscular tension. If your headache, neck, or shoulder pain is coming from your cervical spine, it is called *referred pain*, meaning the pain is coming from an area away from the body party where you feel the pain. So moving or aggravating the cervical spine through maneuvers would cause pain in that referred area. But if you push on the actual

area (i.e., the shoulder blade) and that causes your pain, then you have muscular issues and not pain from your spine.

3. **Strength.** Often the upper back is not as strong as the muscles in the front of the chest. Think about how many more times you have done exercises to strengthen the front of your body compared to your back. Usually people remember doing push-ups and sit-ups instead of upper back strengthening throughout their youth. Lie on your belly with your forehead supported on a rolled towel and your arms at your sides. Can you raise one arm toward the ceiling with your palm facing up? Now move your arm out to the side pointing away from you, palms down. Can you raise it? How about with your arms reaching overhead, palms down? Do this on both sides of the body. If one side feels more difficult to do, there is most likely some muscle imbalance between sides. If you feel strain in your neck as you move your arm, this could indicate muscle imbalance as well.

TREATMENT PLAN

If the tests above indicated a muscle imbalance, do the following:

DAILY STRETCHES

1. *Anterior chest stretch* (E-1)

2. *Chin tucks* (E-8)

3. *Scapular squeeze* (E-2)

4. Gentle rotations of the neck twice a day to increase mobility. Turn your head to the left and right through pain-free range of motion while lying down. While upright, move your neck gently through looking right and left as well as up and down.

SELF-MASSAGE/TRIGGER POINT RELEASE

This can be done every day to give pain relief. Find the sore spots with a tennis ball or foam roller and try to release the trigger points. See the "Myofascial Release" post on www.drdecaria.com under Book Section.

STRENGTHENING

Do every two to three days.

1. *Scapular strengthening series* (E-4)

2. *Yoga cobra pose* (E-7) and *scapular squeeze into locust* (E-3)

The majority of the time, cervical spine and muscular issues are related to positioning throughout the day. Be sure to carefully follow our ergonomic recommendations from Chapter 12. Be sure to take frequent breaks throughout the day to change position, stretch, and move.

PAIN AND/OR NUMBNESS AND TINGLING IN THE ARM? IS IT FROM THE SPINE OR SOMEWHERE ELSE?

Often doctors will tell you that if you have numbness or tingling down your arm, it is coming from a pinched nerve in your neck. Sometimes, even if it is not coming from your neck, your MRI will be abnormal. So how do you know if the symptoms are coming from your neck or a nerve outside of your neck, known as a *peripheral nerve*? Peripheral nerves are nerves that have exited your spine and travel through muscles and little tunnels where they can become compressed and cause pain.

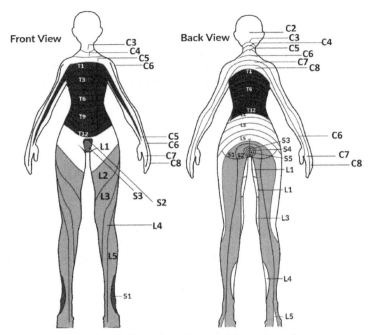

Figure 6. Nerve Root Patterns (dermatomes)

PINCHED NERVE

If you truly have a pinched nerve, your symptoms will follow the pattern of that specific nerve root that is being pinched on your MRI (see Figure 6). An EMG is a test that uses needles and stimulation to look at whether the nerves affected are from a central source (spine) or a peripheral source (nerve outside the spine). These diagnostic test results should all be taken in the context of a history and physical exam, because they can also have results that may not correlate with the area of pain.

Even if all diagnostic tests point to a cervical issue (pinched nerve in neck), I still suggest you run through the rest of this section. We are going to look at three possible sources of peripheral nerve issues that can mimic spine problems but are treated successfully with exercises, behavior modifications, and physical therapy.

PHYSICAL EXAM

1. Sit in a chair with good posture. Look all the way up, all the way down, all the way to the right, and all the way to the left.

2. Tuck your chin back and look up. Then tilt head to left and right (same side ear to same side shoulder).

3. Turn your head to the right about seventy-five percent of the way, look up, and push down on the very top of your head (Figure 7 and Video: *Neck Exam*). Caution: Go slow! Be gentle and easy with your pressure, as this compresses the nerves in your neck. Repeat on the other side. If none of these tests reproduce the shooting pain down your arm in the same pattern as you feel your symptoms, a pinched nerve in your spine is likely not the source, and you should keep reading.

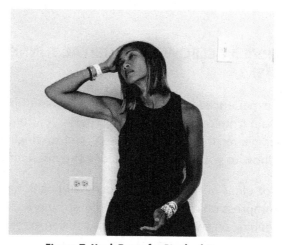

Figure 7. Neck Exam for Pinched Nerve

TREATMENT PLAN

If you do have signs of a pinched nerve, I recommend physical therapy after seeing your physician. If you have any weakness of your arm or hand muscles, I recommend seeing your doctor as soon as possible. They may recommend surgery in certain cases.

PERIPHERAL NERVES THAT MAY BE CAUSING YOUR NECK PAIN

If you found from the above exam that you do not have a pinched nerve from your spine, then continue reading for other possible explanations for your pain. Nerve pain, numbness, and tingling pain can also be caused by issues with peripheral nerves. Peripheral nerves refer to nerves that have exited your spine and are traveling throughout other parts of your body. We will discuss common peripheral nerve pain syndromes below. These issues are often overlooked, as many physicians are quick to diagnose you with a pinched nerve in your neck.

ULNAR NERVE AT ELBOW (I.E., CUBITAL TUNNEL SYNDROME)

We have all experienced bopping our elbow on something and feeling a shooting pain from our "funny bone." That is your ulnar nerve. If it is your ulnar nerve, the pain, numbness, and/or tingling will travel from your elbow to your pinky finger along the inside of your arm.

The causes of ulnar nerve pain are mostly all positional/ergonomic, leading to compression of this nerve. Common culprits are leaning on armrests, sleeping on a very firm mattress causing excess pressure on that area overnight, holding your phone with a bent elbow, or typing with elbows bent for long periods of time.

PHYSICAL EXAM

1. Flex arm to ninety degrees and tap on the inside of your elbow (the side that lines up with your pinky). It should reproduce your symptoms.

2. Keeping your elbows close to your side, bend sharply at the elbow until your palms face the ceiling. This should set off your symptoms down your arm.

TREATMENT PLAN

1. **Exercises:** *Forearm flossing* (E-10). You may feel a reproduction of your symptoms during this, but it should decrease within a few minutes of stopping. Do daily.

2. You can wrap your elbow with foam or a towel, or rest it on a pillow at night. You can also get an elbow brace that will prevent you from bending your elbow too acutely during the day. Some of the topical therapies mentioned in Chapter 17 may help abate symptoms as well.

3. **Tips:** Do not overstretch. Do not massage the actual nerve itself. That will only aggravate it. You can self-massage the muscles between the elbow and wrist, but not the actual nerve in the elbow.

MEDIAN NERVE AT WRIST (I.E., CARPAL TUNNEL SYNDROME OR CTS)

This syndrome is very common. It is caused by excessive pressure on the median nerve as it travels through a tiny tunnel on the inside of your wrist.

Common causes: Compression from repetitive movements, trauma, poor positioning while typing or sleeping, swelling from various physical conditions like pregnancy, or wearing a watch too tight. It is also associated with a variety of systemic diseases.

Symptoms are numbness and tingling in the wrist and hand (typically thumb, pointer, middle, and half of ring finger).

PHYSICAL EXAM

1. You may see muscle wasting of the fat pad at the base of the thumb. Compare one side of the thumb to the other side.

2. You can do a test where you place the back of your hands with wrists in a ninety-degree position with wrist bent and fingers pointing to the ground. Hold this position with your elbows up and straight for sixty seconds. You should get numbness/tingling in your hands. This is the Phalen's test.

3. Another test known as the Tinel's test is to tap directly on the wrist (palm side) and see if it reproduces the numbness/tingling.

TREATMENT PLAN

If these are positive, it points to carpal tunnel syndrome over spine issues.

1. The first step of treatment is a stiff wrist brace for six weeks. Yes, every night. I also suggest wearing it during the day when typing or doing repetitive motions that may trigger the pain.

2. **Exercises:** *Carpal tunnel stretch* (E-9). Do daily.

TENNIS ELBOW OR LATERAL EPICONDYLITIS

This is due to the degeneration of tendons that attach to the bony bump on the outside of your elbow (lateral epicondyle). Often, it is due to muscle strains/imbalances that attach to this bony bump.

PHYSICAL EXAM

1. **Palpate:** Push on the bony bump. If you have pain, it is likely traditional epicondylitis. If you are sore along the forearm muscles that attach, you likely have a strain.

2. **Flexibility/Muscle Tightness Test:** Put both hands directly in front of you at shoulder height and point fingers to ground, palms facing you. Bend wrists as far as you can. If there is an inability to flex at the wrist on the affected side, those muscles are likely tight.

TREATMENT PLAN

1. **Exercises for Forearm Extensors**: As long as it does not aggravate pain, you should do the following exercises five to seven days per week: *Carpal tunnel stretch* (E-9), *scapular strengthening series* (E-4), *tennis elbow eccentric strengthening* (E-11)

GOLFER'S ELBOW OR MEDIAL EPICONDYLITIS

This is elbow pain due to degeneration of tendons that bend the wrist toward the palm of the hand. These tendons are located above the bony bump on the side of the elbow closest to your body (medial epicondyle).

PHYSICAL EXAM

1. **Palpate:** Push on the medial epicondyle/bony bump. See if it reproduces pain. If it does, it is more likely the tendons and not muscles.

2. **Flexibility/Muscle Tightness Test:** Place arms up at shoulder length, palms up to ceiling, and bend wrists down like the carpal tunnel stretch. You should be able to reach a ninety-degree bend on both sides. If one side is significantly tighter, there is tightness of the muscle. Stretches can help with this.

TREATMENT PLAN

1. **Exercises:** *Golfer's elbow eccentric strengthening* (E-12), *scapular strengthening series* (E-4), *carpal tunnel stretch* (E-9), as long as it does not aggravate pain

2. Do five to seven days per week.

For *all* these peripheral nerve issues, E-2 and E-4 will be helpful. Do five to seven days per week.

OTHER CAUSES OF PERIPHERAL NERVE ISSUES

Peripheral nerve issues could be due to a variety of other conditions outside of physical compression of the nerves. These things should be investigated and ruled out: B_{12} deficiency (medications like metformin or proton pump inhibitors for reflux can cause B_{12} deficiency), damage to nerves from chemotherapy agents, or diabetes. These are a few common problems that also cause peripheral nerve damage.

TRUE ROTATOR CUFF TEAR OF SHOULDER?

A rotator cuff tear is a very common finding on a MRI. However, when not associated with trauma, these are rarely pain generators. When a rotator cuff tear happens as a slow degenerative change, it usually is not the cause of your pain and should not require surgery. In these cases, strengthening muscles with the following exercises should alleviate the pain.

WHAT IS THE ROTATOR CUFF?

The rotator cuff consists of four muscles that attach from the shoulder blade to the upper arm: supraspinatus, infraspinatus, teres minor, and subscapularis. These muscles are responsible for stabilizing the shoulder so the arm can move upward and around. If there is a tear in the rotator cuff, raising the arm in front of you or out to the side becomes difficult and painful.

PHYSICAL EXAM

1. First, raise your arms out in front of you with the palms facing down. Then raise them overhead with the palms facing each other.

2. Then raise them to the side, with the palms facing the ground. You may have pain during part of your motion that may go away as the arm approaches overhead.

3. This might indicate the tendon of the rotator cuff is inflamed, getting pinched (impinged), or may have some microtears. This can heal if treated with strengthening exercises, but may lead to a tear with increased pain and decreased range of motion if not.

4. If there is no major loss of motion, you likely do not have a symptomatic rotator cuff tear and should do the exercises below.

TREATMENT PLAN

1. **Exercises:** Stabilizing your shoulder will lead to decreased pain. Do *scapular squeeze* (E-3), *anterior chest stretch* (E-1), *cat/cow* (E-5), and *shoulder strengthening series* (E-6) every other day.

2. Every day, do shoulder range of motion to keep the joint moving. Use your opposite hand to help lift your affected arm and move it through available motions passively. Repeat this ten times, twice a day. See video: *Shoulder Joint Movement*.

DO I REALLY HAVE A LABRAL TEAR OF MY HIP?

So your MRI says you have a labral tear, and you are considering surgery.

Remember, most labral tears are degenerative, meaning they took place over time, and your body has already formed natural defense mechanisms, so the tear itself is not generating pain.

PHYSICAL EXAM

1. Try moving your hip through all the normal range of motions. See video: *Hip ROM*. Compare both sides. The way to tell if it is a labral tear is that the hip will lock during certain movements. This locking can be repetitive and painful. Often, your leg won't move until you shake it or move it in a certain way to release it.

2. If you do not have locking, but an MRI shows a labral tear, you should first try physical therapy (PT) and see if the pain improves through muscular rebalancing.

TREATMENT PLAN

EXERCISES FOR HIP DEGENERATIVE LABRAL ISSUES DUE TO MUSCLE IMBALANCES:

1. Improve your hip range of motion. Place both feet on the ground. Lift one knee up towards your chest, holding your leg either below the knee or under the thigh. Use your hands to guide your hip through all available motions. Do ten times, twice a day. See video: *Hip Joint ROM*.

2. For strengthening, do *bent knee fall out* for stabilization (E-18). Do every other day.

THE LOW BACK

Back pain can be due to a variety of muscular issues—stemming from muscles in the back, legs, buttocks, and even pelvic floor.

We are going to address these one by one to tackle this problem and hopefully avoid unnecessary spine surgeries.

IS MY BACK PAIN MUSCULAR OR FROM MY SPINE?

One confirmatory test is to see if the pain down your leg follows one of the nerve root patterns in Figure 6. If you have pain that only goes down a characteristic nerve root pattern on one or both legs *and* findings on your MRI that support that nerve being compressed, you likely have symptoms from that herniated disc.

Pain from spinal stenosis typically improves when you lean forward, like leaning on a shopping cart. Additionally, you may have leg pain that worsens with walking but improves with rest or leaning forward. This is known as neurogenic claudication. If you are a smoker or former smoker, or have any form of vascular disease, please confirm your doctor has ruled out vascular claudication as a cause of leg pain that worsens with activity and improves with rest. This is an issue with the blood vessels, not the structure of your spine.

If your pain down the leg is only until the knee, you need to consider other causes like facet joint arthritis (little joints in spine) or sacroiliac joint dysfunction, which will be discussed next.

PHYSICAL EXAM

1. If there is a history of trauma, osteoporosis, history of cancer, and/or sudden severe onset of pain, or pain from pushing on the bony protuberances in the middle of your back, it could be a vertebral fracture and should be evaluated in the ER right away for bracing and possible surgical evaluation. If you ever have new severe back pain in the setting of a fever, go to the nearest ER.

2. **Palpate:** This one is easy to assess. If you have localized back pain that you can palpate, and it is about one to two inches to either side of your midline spine, you likely have muscle spasms.

3. If you push midline where your spine is and have pain in that area, or pain that worsens with bending backward or twisting, this could indicate an issue with the tiny joints in your spine (facet joints).

4. **Straight Leg Test**

    a. Lie on your back. Have a partner lift your straight leg to about forty to sixty degrees (about medium-high), and then have them pull your toes toward your head.

    b.   If you have pain down your leg in a similar pattern to what you usually experience, this is a positive straight leg raise test. This tests for dural tension or further proves you may have a nerve root being compressed in your spine.

5. **Posture:** The tilt of your pelvis may give you some information. You can check this standing or lying down with your legs straight.

    a.   If you have a large arch in your lower back, the muscles in the front of your hip (hip flexors and quadriceps) and your lower back may be tight, and the muscles of your glute/hamstring and abdomen may be weak.

    b.   If your lower back is very flat, the muscles in the back of the hip (glutes and hamstrings) may be tight, and your hip flexors, quad, and back muscles may be weak.

    c.   You can confirm/check this with flexibility and strength testing that follows.

6. **Flexibility:**

    a.   Front of the hip: Lying down with your hips at the edge of your bed, bring one knee to your chest and let the other leg drop off the edge of the bed. Then switch sides. Do both legs stretch easily down toward the floor? Can you fully bend your knee to your chest while stretching? If not, the muscles in the front of the leg may be tight.

    b.   Hamstrings: Lying on your back, bring your knee to your chest, then try to straighten your other knee—compare side to side. Is it easy to straighten, or is your leg quite bent? This may indicate tightness in the back of your leg.

7. **Strength:**

    a.   Do strength testing for your legs. You will need a partner to put their hand on you as resistance for each motion (hip movements, knee movements, ankle movements, toe movements). If you find significant differences in your ability to hold against your partner's resistance or pressure, this may indicate involvement of the nerve that innervates that muscle.

b. Muscle imbalances. Often back pain can be caused by muscles around the pelvis/hips and back being "out of balance" (i.e., too tight and/or too weak). We can start to look for these imbalances by checking the flexibility and strength in the hips and back.

c. Compare your left leg to your right leg with the following movements. Do each movement with one leg at a time. Look for differences between the two sides, as well as how easy or hard it is to do each movement. If you have a partner, try to do strength testing against them holding resistance (partner pushing down on your leg in each of these positions while you try to push up against them).

- Lying on your side lifting your top leg to the ceiling

- Lying on your belly lifting one leg off the bed

- Lying on your back lifting one leg toward the ceiling

d. Core/back strength. Lying on your back with your knees bent, can you keep your back flat and pick up one foot (marching). Set that foot down and lift the other. How does that compare side to side? Lying on your stomach, are you able to lift your arms, head, and chest off the floor? This will give you information about how strong your back (and core/abdominal) muscles are (video: *Marching Test*).

8. **Check for a Strained Gluteus Medius**:

a. Low back pain or buttock pain could be a strained gluteus medius. Stand on one leg. If one side is weaker than the other, you will be unable to hold your weight up and will fall to the affected side, or your pelvis may drop on the opposite side. If this is the case, please refer to the piriformis exercises below.

TREATMENT PLAN

If the above exercises determine you have a muscular issue, do the following program.

Exercises: E-13 *child's pose* and E-14 *crescent moon pose* daily.

You should also do the *marching test* as a core strengthening exercise. As an exercise, while doing the march, hold one leg up for one to two seconds, then lower it slowly, and repeat on the other side.

Strengthening Core Exercises: *Marching Video, bent knee fall out* (E-18). Repeat ten times for three sets (thirty marches per leg).

These same exercises can be used if you have a herniated disc, but if the above exam showed you do have one, you should consult with a physical therapist and discuss with them if the McKenzie method will work for you (see Resources). Be mindful that if you are over the age of sixty or have pain upon bending your spine backward while standing, the McKenzie method may not be for you. If it is painful, do not do it.

DO I HAVE TRUE SCIATICA OR PIRIFORMIS SYNDROME?

Many patients present with "sciatica." This refers to pain, numbness, tingling, or shooting pain down the leg, typically down the back of the leg from the buttock. However, if you have this type of pain, it does not always mean the source is your spine. It could be coming from several other causes, one of which is the piriformis muscle. I am going to teach you how to do some tests, so you can tell which one it is.

A herniated disc is typically more common than piriformis syndrome as a cause of shooting pain down the leg. However, sometimes people get the diagnosis of "sciatica" to explain shooting nerve pain down their leg(s), and the presumed source is the spine. However, their pain does not follow the pattern we would expect when we compare their pain pattern on Figure 6 to their MRI report. Just like in the arms, there are peripheral (outside of the spine) nerves that can cause issues.

The sciatic nerve itself is actually the largest and thickest nerve in our bodies. It is formed after nerves from the low lumbar and sacral vertebrae *exit* the spine. They converge and run through the buttocks and down the leg, splitting off into other nerves as they travel.

The piriformis muscle sits deep in your buttock area, and in some people, the sciatic nerve actually runs through it. In others, the sciatic nerve sits under the muscle. So if you have spasms of that muscle, you can have sciatic nerve compression, causing numbness, tingling, or pain down the back of your leg. If you do suffer from piriformis syndrome, then you would have pain or numbness/tingling over the buttock and back of your legs. I have seen some patients have these symptoms simply from always sitting on a thick wallet in their back pocket. Their pain resolved just by removing their wallets (although it does take weeks sometimes for this resolution)! However, if your symptoms are from a nerve compressed by a disc or structure in your spine, it would follow the nerve patterns shown in Figure 6 (i.e., L4, L5, or S1).

Some doctors will say this is not a real syndrome. Yet other doctors, like Dr. Aaron Filler, say this syndrome is so prevalent, the majority of patients with sciatica have it. Dr. Filler found through using MRN (magnetic resonance neurography) that over 93% of cases with sciatica were due to muscular impingement of the nerve.[1] I am not sure the number is that high, but it is certainly a real and prevalent disorder.

SIGNS OF PIRIFORMIS SYNDROME

Usually presents as pain in the buttock, which becomes worse with sitting and may shoot down the back of the leg.

The piriformis is deep in the buttock. You can push deep in the buttock area to find a sore spot or trigger point.

PHYSICAL EXAM

1. Check pelvic height. It could be from gluteus medius strain. If there is a strain, the pelvis rim on the side opposite the strain would be lower.

2. Sit on a chair with your feet flat on the floor. Bring one foot up onto the other knee to do a figure four and see if one side opens up more than the other. If the painful side does not open up as much as the non-painful side, then you need to lengthen and stretch as well as strengthen. If both sides open equally or the affected side opens even more than the unaffected side, then skip the stretching and just do strengthening.

3. Lie on your belly and push up into the cobra pose. If your back or leg pain changes (either improves or worsens), it is more likely coming from a disc or spine issue. If it is from the piriformis, this move will not change your pain.

TREATMENT PLAN

Ironically, even though the muscle feels tight, most of the time the piriformis is actually a lengthened muscle that has developed knots. So it actually needs to be strengthened/shortened to improve. This means that although it is okay to stretch the longer piriformis slightly, do not overdo it. It is okay to stretch once in a while to provide some relief, but do not stretch it excessively. Just gently stretch for short periods of time (thirty seconds maximum).

The massage and stretch techniques below can help give you some temporary relief when it is severe or right before bed to help you sleep. However, the main treatment will be physical strengthening to correct the underlying issue, which is weakness of one side of your gluteal muscles.

Myofascial Release of Piriformis: Place two tennis balls in a sock or one tennis ball on a yoga mat or the floor. Bring foot up to opposite knee in figure four and sit on the ball. You can also use a foam roller. If you cannot get on the floor, you can try against the wall, but it may be hard to get effective release. Once you find a sore spot, sink into it for ten to fifteen seconds.

Exercises: *piriformis stretch* (E-22). Remember, do not overstretch!

Strengthening is the key to recovery. It is usually best to strengthen both hip abductors, as most likely both could benefit from getting stronger. You might find that the stronger side has an easier time completing a set of twenty reps, and you can do this while you are building up to it on your weaker side. The goal is to initially get them to the same strength, so be sure to really focus on the weaker side, doing more reps on that side until it catches up. Once they are equal, continue to strengthen both sides equally.

Exercises: *Hip squeeze* (E-19), *4-way leg lifts* (E-20), *bridge* (E-15). Do every other day.

Positioning Recommendations: Sit with both feet flat on the floor. Don't cross legs. Sleep with a pillow either between your legs if on your side or under your knees if on back. For men, no wallets in back pockets.

IS IT SACROILIAC (SI) JOINT ARTHRITIS?

The sacroiliac joint (SI) is the joint that connects the tail end of your spine to your big pelvic bone. SI joint arthritis can be a tricky diagnosis to make, as it can easily be confused with a pinched nerve from your spine, piriformis syndrome, lumbar facet arthritis, or trochanteric bursitis.

PHYSICAL EXAM

1. From section one, did you find a leg-length discrepancy? Uneven pelvis?

2. To test for SI joint dysfunction, you should refer to the section of this chapter where we examine the two bony protuberances in your back. Are those painful when you push on them? Is your pelvis tilted or hitched up to one side? These could indicate SI joint issues.

3. The next test to see if you have SI joint issues is to lie on your back. Bring your knee all the way up to your chest. That should not cause pain. Then make a figure four with your legs by bringing the foot to the opposite knee and trying to lay your knee flat against the bed (video: *SI Joint Test*). This should cause pain over those bony areas you just felt on your back. You may also experience pain on the outside of the leg or in the groin, but this could indicate possible other causes such as hip bursitis or hip joint osteoarthritis. A physical therapist or pain doctor can help you tell the difference.

TREATMENT PLAN

Remember, the goal of treatment is to return your muscles to their resting state as often as possible. And that takes active effort on your part. No one can do it for you. If your muscles remain weak, you will continue to have pain.

It takes a minimum of three months to see consistent relief, and this is largely dependent on how long your body has been in this state. If muscles have been in a state of tension for many, many years, breaking the cycle will be more challenging.

This joint is commonly affected during pregnancy as well. Support belts are excellent at treating this and should be worn low on the hips, over the two bony areas you palpated earlier. I personally like the OPTP Si-Loc belt or the Serola belt that has extra Velcro straps you can use for added support.

Exercises: *Hip squeeze* (E-19), *pelvic tilt* (E-24), *bridge* (E-15), and *cat/cow* (E-5).

IS THE PAIN ON THE BACK OF MY THIGH COMING FROM MY SPINE OR A STRAINED HAMSTRING?

Sometimes patients will experience pain on the back of their thigh that doctors may attribute to their spine, when the cause is actually a strained hamstring. Let's review how to tell the difference.

PHYSICAL EXAM

1. **Palpate** along the hamstring. See if it is painful. If the source of the pain is your spine, it should not hurt to push on the hamstring.

2. **Strength testing:** To check the strength of your hamstring, while sitting, bend one leg back and have an assistant pull forward. Keep pushing back against their resistance, and don't let the leg straighten. Does this cause pain at your hamstring or behind your knee? If so, it may indicate the hamstring is the problem.

TREATMENT PLAN

1. Exercises
   a. Quad stretch (E-23), calf stretch (E-27)
   b. Strengthen hamstring/glute/hip adductors:
      i. Bridge (E-15)
      ii. Hip squeeze (E-19)
      iii. 4-way hip (E-20)
2. See positioning recommendations under Piriformis section above.

THIGH NUMBNESS

Meralgia paresthetica is a syndrome that is often misdiagnosed as a pinched nerve in the spine. Usually, however, it is due to a nerve being compressed outside the spine at the waist. The lateral femoral cutaneous nerve can be compressed in the groin region from obesity, tight clothing, tight belts, or pregnancy. It can also be caused by trauma and is often seen in diabetics. This syndrome presents itself as burning, tingling, numbness, or pain along the front or outside aspect of the thigh.

This diagnosis is typically made by history alone, as there is no good imaging study for it, and often this is missed on an EMG study because it is such a small nerve. The EMG can be useful, however, to rule out a pinched nerve in the spine. If the EMG comes back as normal, and you have these symptoms, consider this diagnosis.

TREATMENT PLAN

The definitive treatment is behavior modification, including weight loss, wearing loose clothing, avoiding belts, etc. You want to remove the compression on the nerve.

To confirm the diagnosis, you can see an interventional pain doctor who can do an injection of corticosteroid to both diagnose and treat the pain. These injections typically work very well when done in conjunction with the behavior modifications. Nerve pain medications and the supplements discussed at the end of this chapter to support nerve pain can be helpful as well.

A FEW FINAL THOUGHTS ON BACK PAIN/SCIATICA

Point 1: Failed Back Surgery. If you have had back surgery and suffer from persistent back and/or leg pain that radiates down to the knee, you likely have facet joint arthritis or sacroiliac joint issues post spine surgery. I believe many times this comes from the spine surgery altering your spinal structure and furthering muscle imbalances.

These respond well to physical therapy and injections or ablation procedures instead of additional surgeries.

Point 2: Pelvic Floor Dysfunction. If you feel your pain does not fit one of the above categories, if you have onset of back pain during or after a pregnancy, or if you have bladder issues or pain with intercourse, consider seeking a pelvic floor physical therapist. We won't go over these exercises in this book, but a non-relaxed pelvic floor can lead to low back pain and should not be overlooked as a cause. Another thing for new moms to consider is whether they have diastasis recti that is contributing to their low back pain. Diastasis recti is partial or complete separation of your six-pack muscles, or rectus abdominis. If this persists for over three months postpartum, you can see a physical therapist for specific exercises.

HIP PAIN

IS IT HIP JOINT ARTHRITIS OR A MUSCLE/TENDON/BURSITIS?

Many times when patients complain of hip pain, they get a hip X-ray. More often than not, if they are over the age of fifty, there is some degree of arthritis present. For younger patients, MRIs of the hips can sometimes show labral issues that are not the true source of their pain. A lot of the time, pain in the hip is actually stemming from structures that attach to the hip, such as tendons or muscles. These types of pain syndromes respond really well to physical therapy, and it is important to distinguish them before undergoing surgery.

PHYSICAL EXAM

1. Lie flat on your back. Have your partner rotate your leg outward and inward, moving your hip joint. If the joint is the culprit, it will hurt (usually in the groin) to rotate it. You will also have pain with walking that improves with rest.

2. It is important to also see if groin pain is reproduced by pushing on the muscles at the groin. If yes, it may be sartorius, gracilis, or hip adductor muscles. If localized pain, then focus on stretching hip flexors and strengthening hip extensors and abductors.

   Exercises: *Bridge* (E-15), *4-way hip* (E-20). Do every other day. *Psoas stretch* (E-21). Do every day.

3. Gluteus medius strains can lead to hip bursitis and buttock pain. Stand on one foot and then stand on the other foot. If you have a strain, you won't be able to stand easily on the side with the strain. Pain may be on the same side of the strain or opposite.

TREATMENT PLAN

1. If you have a gluteus medius strain, you need to strengthen the gluteal muscles and hip abductors.

   Exercises: *Bridge* (E-15), *glute activator* (E-25).

2. If these are painful, you may need to start with something gentler. See a PT for modifications.

DO I REALLY HAVE A KNEE MENISCUS TEAR OR KNEE LIGAMENT INJURY?

The meniscus is a structure in the knee joint, made of fibrocartilage, that supports pressure in the knee. A meniscal tear usually happens after trauma has occurred. Things that can cause injury to the meniscus are a sudden, excessive straightening of the knee, extreme bending of the knee, or twisting the knee suddenly. Usually these injuries are done in sports, such as skiing.

Meniscal tears are *extremely* common. In fact, a study looking at 991 patients found about sixty percent of those with knee pain had meniscal tears, and about sixty percent of patients without symptoms also had meniscal tears.[2]

SIGNS YOU HAVE A TEAR

You have pain along the knee joint line and not in the back of the knee. Your knee may buckle when you walk up stairs or transition from sitting to standing.

PHYSICAL EXAM

To confirm the diagnosis of a true tear, you need to do a physical exam. With a true tear, you have issues with both passive and active straightening and bending of the knee especially when you add a twist.

1. Stand on one leg with the knee slightly bent. Try turning your trunk to the left and right. If it is impossible or very painful, you may have a tear.

2. Deep squats and "duck walking" will be very difficult if you have a symptomatic meniscal tear. Try these exercises to see if you have a tear.

If your MRI shows a ligament tear but there is no history of trauma or instability of your knee joint, you likely should try to strengthen the muscles above and below the knee joint before proceeding with surgery.

I have seen a number of patients with knee pain have the same imbalance: a tight quad and weak/overstretched hamstring.

TREATMENT PLAN

1. Strengthen around your hip to protect and unload your knee.

2. **Exercises:** *4-way hip* (E-20), *bridge* (E-15), *squats* (E-17 and video). Do every other day.

IS MY KNEE, HIP, SHOULDER JOINT PAIN *REALLY* BONE-ON-BONE ARTHRITIS OR WEAK MUSCLES?

Regardless of what your X-ray says, if you have symptomatic bone-on-bone arthritis, your ability to move (i.e., flex and extend) that joint will be *severely* limited. And when you reach limitations in range of motion, you or your partner should feel bone scraping up against bone.

PHYSICAL EXAM

1. **ROM.** If you have pain and limitation with active ROM but your partner can put you in full or almost full ROM while doing it passively, you need to strengthen your muscles around your joint. If you have limitation of ROM and pain with both active and passive ROM, I still recommend physical therapy before and after surgery, but you likely will benefit from interventional procedures like a Coolief® genicular nerve ablation or a joint replacement.

2. It is important to remember that if you possess normal or near-normal range of motion (regardless of whether the movement itself causes you pain), your bone-on-bone arthritis is not the source of your pain. In most cases, I find a tendon or muscle attached to the joint is strained and this is causing pain. This is likely what happened to my patient earlier who had severe findings on her X-ray but whose symptoms improved with strength training.

TREATMENT PLAN

If the above tests determined you have muscular issues around these joints, try these exercises:

1. **Shoulder**

    a. **Shoulder joint ROM:** Using your opposite hand to help lift your affected arm and move it through available motion passively. See shoulder joint movement video. Do daily.

    b. **Exercises:** *Scapular squeeze* (E-2) and *shoulder series* (E-4). Do every other day.

2. **Knee**

    a. **Exercises:** *Bridge* (E-15), *knee to chest/knee ROM* (E-16), and *4-way hip* (E-20). Do every other day.

3. **Hip**

    a. **Hip ROM:** Bring your leg toward your chest and hold onto your leg, guiding it through its full range of motion by moving it in small circles in both directions (video: *Hip ROM*). Do every day. Exercises: *Hip squeeze* (E-19), *bridge* (E-15), *psoas stretch* (E-21). Do every other day.

IS MY ITB CAUSING ME KNEE OR OUTSIDE THIGH PAIN?

The iliotibial band (ITB) is a thick band of connective tissue that runs from the pelvis across the hip to the knee, that helps to stabilize your joints. Muscles attach into this band. If they are out of balance, the ITB can become tighter, more fibrotic, and put an abnormal pull on the knee and hip.

PHYSICAL EXAM

1. Often a tight ITB will be felt as a click over the outside of the hip or pain at the outer knee with certain movements such as squatting or going up/down stairs.

2. Most ITBs are tender to touch, but you can compare side to side for a difference in tension or sensation.

3. You can also check to see if one ITB is tighter than the other by lying on one side and dropping the top leg back behind the other. With the top leg straight but behind the bottom leg, bend the top leg at the knee and see if it hurts. A tight ITB will be painful with this maneuver. This is a variation of Ober's test.

TREATMENT PLAN (FOR TIGHT ITB)

1. Work on muscle balance around the hip and pelvis.

2. **Exercises:** *Hip squeeze* (E-19) and *4-way hip* (E-20). Do every other day.

IS THE PAIN ON MY OUTSIDE CALF COMING FROM MY SPINE OR SOMETHING ELSE?

The common peroneal nerve travels through the fibular tunnel, which lies on the outside part of your leg, just below the knee. This tunnel is formed by the soleus and peroneus longus muscles. When these muscles strain and thicken, which can happen due to an imbalance or injury, they can impinge on the nerve, causing pain either locally to touch or even down the outside of your calf.

This pain may feel sharp, constant, or throbbing, and some doctors may have told you it is coming from your spine. But for many, it is a result of continuous outward rotation of your feet that is putting excessive pressure on the peroneal muscles.

PHYSICAL EXAM

Try finding the area of your peroneal muscle and push on it. It is a thin muscle on the outside of your lower leg. If this reproduces your pain, it is likely a result of your muscle from poor muscular balance.

TREATMENT PLAN

1. **Exercise:** *Peroneal stretch* (E-28). Do daily.

2. You can also use a muscle roller stick or rolling pin on the peroneal muscle to release the trigger points, and topical therapies described in Chapter 17 for relief.

WHAT IS CAUSING MY ANKLE PAIN?

It is crucial to check for imbalances in the hips and pelvis as foot and ankle pain is usually a sign of an issue higher up, such as a strained or weak gluteus medius muscle. Please refer to these sections and do whatever exercises are appropriate.

If you have been told you have ankle arthritis, you should have loss in the range of motion of your ankle, not just pain with moving your ankle. The posterior tibialis and peroneal muscles, as well as tendons around your ankle, can often cause pain. These will respond to strengthening techniques.

An ankle fusion is a surgery done for arthritis that really affects how you walk, leading to further imbalances, so be sure to do a full evaluation with a physical therapist prior to surgery. They can guide you on specific exercises.

PHYSICAL EXAM

You can palpate the muscles around the ankle and see if those are causing pain versus moving the joint itself.

TREATMENT PLAN

If you have ankle pain, doing daily *calf stretches* (E-27) can help.

FOOT PAIN

Patients are often told their pain is due to a bone spur or another condition found on an X-ray when, in fact, it is due to imbalances triggering plantar fasciitis or tendonitis in the foot. Often, symptoms can be tied to a fallen arch that has occurred due to muscle weaknesses higher up in the chain. The fallen arch then causes other issues.

PHYSICAL EXAM

When standing, have someone take a picture or examine your arches. If they are flat, either on one side or both, consider doing these exercises to help with painful issues in your feet.

TREATMENT PLAN

1. **Exercises:** *Tripod foot posture* (E-29) and *toe curls* (E-30). Do every day.

2. In Chapter 12, we go over the importance of footwear, which can greatly help foot pain. A podiatrist and physical therapist can help.

ADDITIONAL TIPS FOR THOSE SUFFERING

NERVE PAIN SUPPLEMENTS

If you suffer from nerve pain (pain that shoots in a nerve distribution [Figure 6] and/or numbness/tingling/burning sensations), you are likely to benefit from the following supplements: alpha-lipoic acid, CoQ10, and acetyl-L-carnitine. My personal favorite is alpha-lipoic acid, as it is a powerful antioxidant, and studies have shown it to reduce nerve damage and improve nerve pain.[3,4] You can read more about these supplements, and others for various pain conditions, in Chapter 11.

MASSAGE

As the majority of people suffering from chronic pain actually have muscular issues, you are likely to find relief from physical therapy and massage therapists. In some cases, chiropractic adjustments can help as well, particularly in the setting of low back pain. Be sure to discuss with your doctor that it is safe to undergo adjustments and check the credentials of who you are seeing. I also advise following personal recommendations from other patients who have had similar conditions to yours and been treated successfully by a given practitioner.

ACUPUNCTURE

Acupuncture has also been shown by many National Institutes of Health (NIH) studies to be effective for headaches, epicondylitis, fibromyalgia, muscle pain, arthritis, low back pain, and carpal tunnel syndrome. Be sure to check the training of who you see because not all acupuncturists practice true acupuncture. Some use acupuncture needles for dry needling, which can also be effective for muscle pain in the way trigger point injections can be, but it is a very different approach.

Be sure to find an acupuncturist that is licensed, board-certified, and went to an accredited program. Be sure to check with your insurance plan, as sometimes acupuncture is covered. If after four to five treatments you are not seeing some sort of benefit beyond the treatment day itself, it is time to re-evaluate whether acupuncture is the right treatment for you. You can discuss with your acupuncturist, functional medicine practitioner, or pain doctor.

BARNES' MYOFASCIAL RELEASE THERAPY

Barnes' Myofascial release therapy is a type of manual massage therapy that I believe is more effective than a traditional massage for pain. The technique involves longer holds to help to release the fascia in your system. This can greatly help muscle imbalances and chronic pain. The Resources section has additional information on finding a provider. Be sure to check with your insurance carrier, as this is sometimes covered by insurance if you have a prescription.

FOR THOSE STILL IN PAIN

If you do these exercises for forty-five days and your pain has not significantly improved, make sure you read the other sections of Part 1.

CHAPTER 5

MIND–BODY PAIN SYNDROME: UNDERSTANDING THE LINK

*"There's nothing like a little physical pain
to keep your mind off your emotional problems."*
—Dr. John Sarno

Frank is a forty-nine-year-old schoolteacher and father of two teenage children. He came to my clinic after suffering an exacerbation of his low back pain. It was so bad that he had to take multiple days off work, exceeding his paid time off. He reported symptoms of central back pain all day long, severe soreness upon waking, an inability to get out of bed, poor sleep, and a fifteen-pound weight gain over the past month. He had a history of mild degenerative disk disease (arthritis) on multiple spine levels on a recent lumbar MRI, along with two small mild disc bulges. He had met with surgeons in the past, but until recently, none had recommended surgery. The one he met with a few weeks prior had said he could potentially do surgery, but the outcome was uncertain. He had about a fifty percent chance of success. After Frank heard this, the pain significantly worsened. It now shot down both legs and became so severe he could not leave his bed.

I dug a bit deeper and discovered that the onset of his pain correlated with the start of the school year. On top of that, his wife had been pressuring him recently about their limited finances, as she wanted them to buy a house. He told me he was overwhelmed at the idea of a mortgage, since they were barely able to make rent payments, and he did not have a good credit history.

I asked him if he had ever heard of tension myositis syndrome, a term coined by Dr. John Sarno. He had not, and I told him I thought that was his diagnosis. I instructed him to read Dr. Sarno's book, *Healing Back Pain*, with an open mind and to follow up with me in a week.

At first, he was skeptical about the idea that his pain came from stress alone. Understandably so, as every other doctor had told him something was wrong with his back. We worked closely, doing worksheets to break through some of the misconceptions he had about his pain—addressing fears that he had injured himself at work and erasing the label of degenerative disc disease that he had grown attached to. He began to understand that there was actually nothing structurally wrong with his back and that he was going to heal. He started journaling, along with swimming twice a week.

It did not take long for his pain to dissipate. Within three months, his pain had disappeared. He continued to follow up with me periodically before major life events, having some internal fears that the pain would return, even though he knew it was related to stress. His pain never flared again.

If you are experiencing thoughts of hurting yourself or others, please call 911 and seek care from the nearest emergency room. These types of thoughts should not be managed alone. Doctors and medications can truly help you in this stage.

You can also call the Suicide Hotline 24 hours a day at 1-800-273-8255.

YOUR DOCTOR DOESN'T KNOW WHY YOU'RE IN PAIN

Pain is the number one reason patients go to the doctor. And the overwhelming majority of the time, the doctor does not have a cure but will give you a diagnosis and hand you a pill. They might tell you that there's nothing major going on, or that maybe it's muscle pain or old age. Old age does not cause pain. There are many people over the age of seventy living without pain and many under thirty living in daily pain.

You may be thinking that I'm about to tell you the pain is in your head and that if you just think it away, it will disappear. That is not true. Your pain is real; it *is* physical, but it is tied to a deep mind–body connection. You are in this chapter because the structural issues found on your physical exam and imaging reports have not shown a condition that supports how severe your pain is. Maybe you had surgery and the scar has healed but you continue to have pain. This surprises your doctors, and they tell you the fusion looks great on X-ray, but you're still miserable. Or maybe you have some abnormalities on your MRI, but the pinched nerve the doctor sees does not correlate with your pattern of pain.

You are here because most medical treatments have either failed to cure your pain or only partially improved it. This chapter is for those of you who do not have structural causes that completely explain how much pain you are in.

As in all types of pain, we are looking to find the source to heal your pain, and in the case of Mind-Body Pain Syndrome (MBPS), the source is in the mind, even though the pain felt in the body is real. This type of pain is difficult to treat and frustrating to experience. I feel deeply for those who suffer from mind–body syndrome. Don't lose hope. There are ways to heal.

BIOLOGY OF PAIN

While pain can be felt in all areas of the body, the decision to actually interpret that signal as "pain" lies within your brain and brainstem.

Your brainstem is like a circuit board that regulates your blood vessels, heart rate, breathing, and digestive tract. It also regulates pain by projecting signals from your brain back through your spinal cord. Although we focus so much on treating pain by treating the various body parts, the key often lies in treating the brain. The brain decides if what just happened to your body will be interpreted as pain.

I understand this may be very confusing because as a society, we have grown accustomed to attributing pain to structural damage. We think that if our foot hurts, the problem lies solely in something that injured our foot. The reality is the majority of patients in chronic pain do not actually show signs of tissue damage in their bodies. An example of this is fibromyalgia. Often patients with fibromyalgia are told all their lab and imaging studies are normal. However, the pain these individuals experience *is* real.

Chronic pain truly is a vicious cycle to some unlucky individuals. When you break a bone, you have an acute injury and acute pain. But the fracture, as well as your pain, should heal within weeks to months. However, sometimes, despite the fracture healing, some individuals are left suffering from chronic pain, while others recover completely. Why? Because a cycle of chronic pain has begun in their nervous system. In some patients, the ongoing pain is perpetuated by a muscle weakness (a physical issue), and for others, a heightened level of mental stress is the recurring source of injury. For millions of unlucky individuals, their brains have turned on the pain cycle.

MISSING THE MIND AS A SOURCE OF PAIN

Many medical doctors and scientists who study and treat pain consider the experience primarily a physical phenomenon. That is what is taught to conventional doctors in medical school.

Let's go back in time a bit. For thousands of years, pain was seen as secondary to an injury in the body. In the 1960s, two scientists, Melzack and Wall,[1] discovered that our pain receptors, or nociceptors, are actually in our brain and spinal cord, and not on whatever area of the body was injured. These nociceptors signal our brain when the nerve cells in the skin or internal organs detect something causing damage. This protective phenomenon is what leads our brains to make us yank our hand away from a hot stove after we touch it.

Melzack and Wall made another interesting observation. They identified that pain is a complex phenomenon and a highly subjective state. In other words, pain is largely affected by factors such as emotions, one's previous experiences, and cultural beliefs, in addition to the sensory input described by the body (after we touch that hot stove).

Even the International Association for the study of pain (IASP) has defined pain as

"an unpleasant sensory and emotional experience associated with actual or potential tissue damage, or described in terms of such damage."[2] The key word being "potential" tissue damage.

Over time, we have seen remarkable stories of severe injury causing no pain (wounded soldiers on the battlefield), as well as patients with no injury and severe pain (fibromyalgia).

As Melzack and Wall explained, psychological factors such as one's cultural and emotional state can heighten or lessen the pain signal before it registers in higher brain centers, which leads to our perception of pain.[3] What this means is that two individuals can touch the same hot stove, but based on their emotional state, their brains will decide how their body will interpret the severity of the pain.

Even more interesting is the fact that many cases of chronic pain seem to occur without any direct trauma or tissue damage at all.[4] And if tissue damage is not needed to stimulate these pain emotional centers in the brain, we can conclude that pain can result from both physical and psychological injury. That is, a severe emotional trauma, such as the loss of one's parent, can be the "injury" that leads to chronic pain.

A PICTURE IS NOT WORTH A THOUSAND WORDS

X-rays, CT scans, and MRIs have been used as diagnostic tools for years but often provide diagnoses that do not correlate with pain. *The New York Times* published an article in 2008 titled "The Pain May Be Real, but the Scan Is Deceiving," which examined this concept in detail. The article discusses the high incidence of "abnormal" imaging findings in patients with no pain.

Despite knowing this, in the last twenty-two years, we have ordered billions of dollars' worth of additional (and often worthless) imaging studies in the pursuit of finding a diagnostic label to attach to a painful symptom.

For example, patients presenting with non-specific low back pain may get a lumbar X-ray. Occasionally, these X-rays provide important pathologies, but more often than not, they have a long list of findings that are unrelated to one's symptoms. Some of these findings involve frightening words such as transitional vertebra, spina bifida occulta, and spondylolysis. These are congenital abnormalities in bony structure that are often blamed for pain, but—despite their scary-sounding names—most of the time do not cause pain.[5] And whether a lumbar X-ray is normal or abnormal, the majority of patients with back pain will go on to get an MRI scan—a test that can cost anywhere from $400 to $2,500.

A study by Jarvik[6] showed that not only are MRI scans for low back pain leading to a wide array of pathological "labels" for the patient, but also these do not demonstrate improvement in outcomes. The authors argue patients suffer from these labels since they may modify activities to "protect" their damaged spines, which can lead to them developing other issues.

This is true for many body parts, not just the back. Often, imaging findings are normal age-related changes and do not signify painful conditions. For example, only fifty percent of people with X-ray evidence of knee osteoarthritis (the wear-and-tear type of arthritis) even have pain.[7]

WHERE THE BODY MEETS THE BRAIN: THE WORK OF DR. SARNO

There is no way to talk about Mind-Body Pain Syndrome without mention of the greatest contributor to this movement, Dr. John Sarno. Dr. Sarno coined the term *tension myositis syndrome* (TMS). TMS is a Mind-Body Pain Syndrome.

Dr. Sarno defined TMS as a painful disorder due to "oxygen deprivation to muscles, nerves, tendons, and ligaments." He felt this oxygen deprivation was the "direct result of specific emotional situations." He refers in his books to a study by Fassbender and Wegner. This study reported microscopic findings of oxygen deprivation from muscle biopsies in patients with back pain.[8]

Although this concept has not been widely studied since or replicated in large-scale trials, we certainly have common conditions where we see oxygen deprivation causing muscle pain. Myocardial ischemia, for example, is the cause of heart attacks and abnormal heart rhythms. Myocardial ischemia occurs when blood flow through blood vessels to your heart is reduced, preventing the heart muscle from receiving enough oxygen. This ischemia, or lack of oxygen, causes the muscle pain, or chest pain, often felt by patients during heart attacks. Dr. Sarno believed that oxygen deprivation to muscles of the back was the root cause of most people's back pain. He felt patients that are highly tense and anxious get oxygen deprivation to their neck and back muscles, resulting in pain.

What Dr. Sarno describes in his books are large numbers of patients with normal physical exams yet abnormalities on imaging studies.[9,10] These patients had severe pain that was not attributable to anything structural (i.e., the findings on their MRI did not explain their pain). He felt a number of commonly diagnosed MRI findings, such as herniated disc, spondylolysis, spinal stenosis, and scoliosis, were never the cause of physical pain. His theory was based on the number of studies demonstrating that people with no pain have these findings just as frequently as people with pain. There are numerous studies that have shown this.[11,12]

There is limited research specifically on TMS. There was one study I came across by Dr. Schechter on fifty-one patients in his clinic who underwent TMS treatment.[13] The patients all had low back pain with no structural pathology and normal physical exams. These patients were treated with a cognitive therapy program (a thought-restructuring program). Their results showed around fifty percent of subjects improved.

In his book *Mind Over Back Pain*, Dr. Sarno reports the results of a survey he conducted on one hundred of his patients with TMS. Sixty percent had gradual onset of TMS with no attributable physical injury. He saw this as an indicator that their pain could not be physical in nature, and found that once they identified and accepted that the pain was triggered by emotions, they recovered. He recommended patients who have pain that began without any sort of physical trauma look at possible emotional links and stressors that were taking place around that time, as they may suffer from TMS.

To many, Dr. Sarno's work is still seen as controversial. One criticism of Dr. Sarno's work was the lack of scientific data and the reliance largely on results he witnessed with his own patients. No large controlled scientific trials were conducted on his method, either by him or others. In the medical world, the lack of large scientific trials makes someone's work merely "anecdotal" and less likely to be accepted into conventional medical care.

However, he published books and taught other practitioners based on his own experience with patients he had successfully treated. Despite the lack of scientific trials, his anecdotal data is quite impressive, and his work has helped heal thousands of lives. The stories of practitioners who treat patients in a similar fashion to Dr. Sarno, such as Dr. Howard Schubiner and Dr. David Schechter, are impressive as well.[14] You can find out more information in the Resources section.

CHEMICAL IMBALANCES TRIGGER MIND-BODY PAIN SYNDROME

To understand Mind-Body Pain Syndrome (MBPS) better, we need to dig further into the science. When faced with stressful situations, our bodies go into a fight-or-flight response, activating our sympathetic nervous system (SNS). This response, which causes our heart rate to increase, our breathing rate to increase, and our muscles to tense, is what equips us to deal with an attack. Our ancestors would have this response when hunting or encountering predators. However, when the stressor would pass, their bodies would return to a relaxed (parasympathetic) state. We are designed so that our bodies should remain primarily in this relaxed state, with only occasional activation of our fight-or-flight system. Unfortunately, our bodies are not designed to be able to handle states of constant stress.

Stress targets specific areas in our brain. The hippocampus is a part of our brain that supports memory and mood and is a target of stress hormones. The amygdala, which is the part of our brain that detects and responds to threats in our environment, as well as the prefrontal cortex play a role in decision-making and regulating our emotions. They also control our hormonal, autonomic, and neuroendocrine functions. In other words, these areas of the brain are involved chemically in our stress response.[15]

Stress is not always bad. Stressful experiences trigger the release of hormones that produce a response in our hippocampus, hypothalamus, and other brain regions. These effects can be both adaptive (helpful) and maladaptive (damaging). For example, stress can be helpful by enabling us to run from an intruder, but it can also cause negative effects such as preventing us from getting a good night's sleep.

Overcoming stressful experiences can lead to personal growth, adaptation, and the development of skills needed to be resilient in the future. Unfortunately, the way our brain interprets some stressful experiences, in addition to an inability to turn stress off, can lead to a proliferation of negative health sequences and symptoms, such as high blood pressure or heart disease.

When you are constantly in a state of arousal and stress, your body struggles to keep your hormones and chemicals in check. The constant stress leads to problems with the hypothalamic-pituitary-adrenal (HPA) axis, the part of our body responsible for regulating these chemicals and hormones. This dysregulation has been shown to lead to chronic pain and chronic fatigue.[16]

Fibromyalgia and temporomandibular disorders are two pain conditions that have been linked to higher baseline sympathetic (fight-or-flight) system activity, particularly at night, and lower baseline parasympathetic (resting) activity. Since our resting system is designed to counterbalance our fight-or-flight system and bring us back to a resting state, the goal is to spend the majority of our day in the resting state. Patients with Mind-Body Pain Syndrome (MBPS) live mostly in the fight-or-flight state.

A key hormone driving chronic pain is cortisol. Cortisol is our fight-or-flight hormone. In high-stress individuals, studies have found physical symptoms of pain increase due to issues with cortisol levels. Chronic stress and the subsequent increase on your body's cortisol levels lead to increased sensitivity to painful stimuli and a higher incidence of mood disorders.[17]

The good news is that the effects of this continuous stress on the brain is not irreversible. Your brain is amenable to recovery, restructuring behaviors, and interventions that include therapy, medications, and changes in lifestyle factors that positively impact your body. Studies have shown exercise, dietary changes, and improved social support systems can favorably restructure the effects of stress on your brain tissue.[18]

The most important thing to remember is you can make changes to affect your resilience to stressful situations and also change your neuroplasticity, or brain chemistry, in a favorable way. We are going to learn how to do that in this chapter.

MIND–BODY DIAGNOSES IN MAINSTREAM MEDICINE

Despite the controversy surrounding acceptance of Mind-Body Pain Syndrome (MBPS), Western conventional medicine has plenty of evidence to support that there are diseases where the mind causes physical symptoms. These diagnoses are known as *somatoform disorders*: a group of disorders where mental or psychiatric conditions cause physical pain symptoms.

The *DSM-V* (*Diagnostic and Statistical Manual of Mental Disorders*) is produced by the American Psychiatric Association and is utilized by conventional medical doctors to classify certain mental illnesses. They have strict criteria to meet certain diagnoses. Before I dive into what a somatoform disorder is, I want to note that many of my patients with MBPS would not meet this criterion. However, I am describing these conditions so you understand that conventional medicine does accept that the mind can generate physical symptoms without an attributable physical cause.

To meet the criteria for a somatoform disorder, one must have high levels of anxiety and/or mood symptoms accompanying physical pain symptoms. They describe pain symptoms in the extremities, head, abdomen, joints, back, joints, chest, and rectum, as well as during menstruation, during sexual intercourse, or during urination.

These pain syndromes coexist with gastrointestinal symptoms, sexual symptoms, and some neurological symptoms (such as impaired balance, localized weakness, and loss of sensation). These symptoms take place in systems in our body that are affected by changes in our sympathetic nervous systems (SNS).

There is a long list of criteria that must be met in order to have a medically-defined diagnosis of a somatoform disorder. Many of my patients do not meet criteria for these disorders. However, I believe that MBPS is a much more minor form of somatoform disorder that presents as pain complaints, typically in the neck, back, hips, or feet. It is triggered by anxiety, previous or current emotional traumas, and/or unresolved tensions.

HIGH PREVALENCE OF MIND-BODY PAIN SYNDROME

Despite the fact that diagnoses of somatoform disorders are relatively infrequent due to the extreme criteria needing to be met to obtain the diagnosis, Mind-Body Pain Syndrome (MBPS) is highly prevalent. Scientific journals have shown that up to fifty percent of primary care visits are with patients displaying physical symptoms that cannot be explained by a physical or medical condition.[19] Fifty percent! Since the majority of the time these patients do not meet the psychiatric criteria for the somatoform disorders above, many of these people leave their doctor's offices with no diagnosis and maybe a prescription for physical therapy or a recommendation to take some ibuprofen.

However, some researchers have coined a term to explain this phenomenon: *somatic preoccupation.* Somatic preoccupation has long been described in the medical literature and refers to those with unexplained physical symptoms that appear to be tied to emotions.[20]

Multiple studies show that patients with unexplained physical symptoms tend to have coexisting mental illnesses, such as anxiety and mood disorders.[21]

Unfortunately, many times, conventional medical doctors dismiss these patients or don't believe they are telling the truth because they can't tie their symptoms to a structural or metabolic issue. This leads to further anxiety and continues to drive the syndrome. By not identifying the syndrome appropriately, patients are not receiving the care they need, and this further propagates their pain cycle.

A number of studies have demonstrated that having clinically significant but unexplained physical symptoms leads to increased stress, excessive preoccupation with one's symptoms, inaccurate beliefs about what is causing these symptoms, and costly, unnecessary imaging studies and treatment efforts.[22,23,24,25] Unfortunately, this heightened anxiety drives MBPS symptoms even further.

I hope that as we learn more about the power of the mind, these negative patient experiences are more infrequent and MBPS is more commonly detected and diagnosed.

IDENTIFYING MIND-BODY PAIN SYNDROME

To help better identify if you have Mind-Body Pain Syndrome (MBPS), the list below includes symptoms, common diagnoses, and key life events that I have seen often coexist in MBPS patients. These conditions are found in individuals with an overactive sympathetic nervous system, which serves as a risk factor to developing MBPS.

PAIN CONDITIONS COMMONLY CAUSED BY MBPS

Abdominal pain
Bladder pain
Carpal tunnel syndrome
Cubital tunnel syndrome
Chronic fatigue syndrome
Complex regional pain syndrome (CRPS)
Gastrointestinal disorders (IBS, IBD)
Fibromyalgia
Foot pain (Achilles tendon, sesamoiditis, toe arthritis)
Headaches (migraines, tension, occipital)
Irritable bladder syndrome (interstitial cystitis)
Myofascial pain syndrome
Neck and back pain
Pelvic pain
Piriformis syndrome
Tendonitis
TMJ (temporomandibular joint syndrome)
Whiplash

SYMPTOMS COMMONLY TIED TO MBPS

Acid reflux/heartburn
Abdominal pain
Constipation or diarrhea
Headaches
Anxiety
Depression
Rashes/hives
Muscle pain
Joint pain

PAST EXPERIENCES COMMONLY TIED TO MBPS

Death of loved one
Divorce or separation of parents
Divorce or separation in your own relationship
Emotional abuse (past or present)
Physical abuse (past or present)
Sexual abuse (past or present)
Caring for sick children, sick relatives, or aging parents
Financial stressors

HOW AN OVERACTIVE SYMPATHETIC NERVOUS SYSTEM LEADS TO PHYSICAL PAIN

Many of the stressors faced by our ancestors are no longer issues for us. We have food readily available at the click of a button or from a quick grocery store run. We no longer have predators chasing us through the fields. The days of hunting and gathering as a means for survival are long gone.

Yet many of us spend the majority of our day in sympathetic nervous system (SNS) overdrive due to modern-day stressors. Interpersonal relationship struggles; physical, emotional, or sexual trauma; financial stressors; work deadlines; and even things such as holding ourselves to high social standards via social media. This puts us in a state of constant stress, particularly type A (high achieving, competitive, anxious) individuals.

So rather than living in a state of rest the majority of the day, with short bursts of fight-or-flight overdrive, the converse is actually taking place. When we live in a state of chronic stress, we continuously remain in the fight-or-flight state. Our sympathetic systems are working overtime. When the stressors we face are either traumatic enough or continue nonstop, they start to cause health issues. One of these is physical pain.

When we are constantly activating our sympathetic nervous system, we release hormones in our body that result in a vicious cycle of muscle tension and even gastrointestinal (GI) tract and urinary tract spasms. These spasms can be terribly painful and present as irritable bowel syndrome or interstitial cystitis (a painful bladder syndrome).

The chemicals responsible for this response are cortisol, sympathetic and parasympathetic transmitters, cytokines, and metabolic hormones. The pain arises when our body cannot regulate and rebalance these hormones, a state known as hypothalamic-pituitary-adrenal (HPA) axis dysregulation.

There are numerous animal studies from Italy that demonstrate that our SNS controls our muscle spindles.[26,27,28] Muscle spindles are small capsular-shaped structures responsible for our movement. In other words, our fight-or-flight stress response is directly tied to our muscles.

Since those studies, Walt McNulty and practitioners at Sharp Memorial Hospital in San Diego have studied the role of mental stress in the development of chronic muscle pain.[29]

McNulty's group investigated muscles with trigger points (palpable, taut areas of muscle) versus muscles without trigger points. They found the trigger points, on a microscopic level, have muscle spindles that are regulated by our fight-or-flight response (sympathetic nervous system). In other words, after inducing psychological or emotional stress, the trigger point, or sore muscle, became stimulated. The reason this happens is because the muscle spindle itself carries pain chemicals and receptors (substance P and unmyelinated C fibers). Both of these are key parts of the body's pain pathways.[30] In other words, the emotional stress triggers activation of this muscle spindle within the muscle itself, which causes pain in that person on a chemical level.

Sonia Banks did the same study but added relaxation.[31] The trigger points became activated during stress, but then decreased during relaxation periods. This lends support to the fact that relaxing the mind can relax your painful muscle spasms.

Even more interesting, studies at Sharp Memorial Hospital in San Diego looked specifically at type A individuals. They referred to them as "internalizers," people who are self-critical, anxious perfectionists. This group of eighty type A graduate students had more pain in their muscle trigger points when anxious than they did during periods of no anxiety.[32]

You may have felt that periods of stress in your life have aged you. Scientific data actually supports that notion. Studies have found that chronic stress causes malfunctioning of your stress hormone regulation pathway and can accelerate the aging of your brain.[33] This takes place due to excessive amounts of cortisol, sympathetic activity, and proinflammatory cytokines, along with a decline in parasympathetic activity. Luckily, scientists have shown that this shrinkage of brain tissue due to stress is reversible with the right therapy. This chapter may even help you anti-age your brain!

OUR EMOTIONS CAN IMPACT OUR PERCEPTION OF PAIN

You have likely already experienced psychosomatic pain in your life. Perhaps you had a belly ache when you were nervous or headaches on a very stressful day. These are all physical manifestations of emotions.

Luckily, functional neuroimaging techniques have been developed that allow scientists to study the brain effects of various emotional states and how they may impact pain and pain perception.

Scientists have come to understand that the anterior cingulate gyrus is a part of our brain that makes us feel physical pain.[34] They have also discovered that this same area can be triggered by harmful psychological stimuli—things that threaten the emotional well-being of a person, such as the loss of a child or the pain of depression.

Let's take a look at an example. A study looked at subjects playing a video ball-tossing game, while monitoring their brains on a functional MRI. A functional MRI is a live imaging study that takes a snapshot of what is happening in various parts of the brain. When the individuals were excluded from the game, they experienced distress from the emotional rejection. This distress correlated with increased blood flow to the physical pain parts of the brain (the anterior cingulate gyrus and insular cortices). Interestingly, they found the pattern of blood flow to these areas of the brain was the exact same as if the subjects had been stuck with a needle. They also found the greater the social distress, the more active these pain centers became.[35] If the pain centers became active with this scenario, imagine what would happen if someone underwent a divorce or was bullied at school?

Dr. Gundel and his group did studies on grieving individuals and produced the same results. Whether triggered by grief or depression, or a broken bone or spinal cord injury, the biological process of initiating the pain cycle appears to be the same.[36] And when the grief and pain is ongoing, or the depression and anxiety ineffectively treated, this continuous input triggers a vicious cycle of pain. Your body grows accustomed to triggering these pathways due to years of negative emotions, and eventually these can transfer into physical symptoms.

In fact, studies have demonstrated that simply looking at pictures that elicit emotional pain can result in physical pain. A researcher, Shimo, and his group conducted a study in 2011 where eleven patients with back pain were shown a picture of a painful experience (a man carrying luggage in a crouched position) while monitoring their brains with a functional MRI. What they found was that one hundred percent of the patients with a history of low back pain reported discomfort when shown the picture. Additionally, a number of areas in the cortex became activated that are involved in our pain sensation pathways, including the insula, supplementary motor area, premotor area, thalamus, pulvinar, posterior cingulate cortex, hippocampus, fusiform, gyrus, and cerebellum.[37]

Studies have also shown that back pain levels are higher when one is anxious or angry.[38] For example, a study demonstrated that showing subjects a picture of an ex-girlfriend, or triggering feelings of social rejection, lit up both emotional and physical pain pathways in the brain.[39] After seeing these pictures, the subjects experienced pain.

Interestingly, studies have shown that individuals who suppress emotions exhibit higher pain levels.[40] Scientists have found that the suppression of emotions—which is often done by victims of physical, emotional, or sexual abuse—causes an even greater level of pain than those suffering other emotional triggers. Expressing emotions is key to recovery for those suffering from emotional pain. It is detrimental to bury your emotions and this may be a reason you have not yet broken your pain cycle.

The fact that scientists have proven that pathways in the brain tied to pain are also tied to emotion provides further proof that prolonged pain conditions may be tied to emotional conditions. Pain can be triggered by memories of unpleasant experiences, repression of these unpleasant experiences, or current stressors/unpleasant emotions.

WHEN YOUR BRAIN IS PRIMED FOR PAIN: HOW THE CYCLE BEGINS

We have described on a scientific level that stress hormones can cause pain and emotions are tied to pathways that trigger pain, but why does this lead to a cycle of chronic physical pain in some individuals but not others?

The way our brain processes emotions impacts if and when these negative emotions lead to physical pain. Some bodies are primed from past traumas and a trigger will tip them into pain. For others, pain develops over time due to living in a state of continuous stress. We will review the various risk factors one by one.

In my experience, patients suffering MBPS vary in the severity of their symptoms based on the severity of their triggering cause. Those who have suffered from major traumas, particularly in childhood, or post-traumatic stress disorder (PTSD) are the most challenging to treat.

IMPORTANCE OF CHILDHOOD TRAUMAS

I want you to take a moment and reflect on your childhood. Was it pleasant? Were there any traumatic moments? Perhaps you were bullied, your parents got divorced, your family struggled financially, or you were the victim of abuse?

Anxiety and social stress early in life and during adulthood have powerful pain initiating and amplifying effects. For decades, science has shown a relationship between trauma and chronic pain.

It is no mystery that stress in childhood can trigger health issues. Emotional experiences in childhood get imprinted in the amygdala, the emotion center of our brain. Children growing up in emotionally cold families have been shown to have poorer mental and physical health later in life.

Abuse in childhood is a well-known risk factor for depression, post-traumatic stress disorder, chronic pain disorders of unknown cause, substance abuse, and even diabetes and heart disease.[41]

Animal studies have shown infants with stressful environments have overly active autonomic nervous systems.[42] Those exposed to abuse have repeatedly been shown to have a high likelihood of developing chronic pain.[43] Childhood traumas have been associated with abnormalities within the control board that keeps our hormones in check (the hypothalamic-pituitary-adrenal axis). Problems with this "hormonal control board" predispose people to developing chronic pain later in life.[44]

CASE STUDIES: TRAUMA AND PAIN

There is significant overlap between Mind-Body Pain Syndrome and Central Pain Syndrome.[45,46,47] This concept is discussed more in Chapter 7 and is particularly relevant to those who have suffered childhood trauma. Such trauma creates biochemical imbalances and alters nervous systems so that victims of trauma are primed to develop Mind-Body and Central Pain Syndromes. Sometimes, because they have been primed, it can be a seemingly unrelated or innocuous emotional stress or a minor physical injury that throws them into an unrelenting mind–body pain cycle.

IMPACT OF ABUSE

I took care of a forty-two-year-old female with back pain that started when she was changing jobs. Although it was not a particularly stressful transition, it was still a change, and she experienced anxiety leading up to it. Her back pain started in the few days leading up to the job change. She did not relate the two events to each other because she was happy with her new position, and her back pain remained unchanged. What we later discovered was that she had been the victim of child abuse from her uncle and that her mother had never believed her. These two horrific childhood traumas had primed her system to be set up for the development of Mind-Body Pain Syndrome (MBPS) at some point in her life, and her mildly stressful job change was the trigger. She improved significantly with biofeedback and other approaches to cognitive therapy, including expressing her thoughts and emotions surrounding these events for the first time in her life.

Those suffering from traumas likely need a combination of talk therapy and pain-specific psychotherapy (i.e., biofeedback and cognitive behavioral therapy). These will be discussed in more detail at the end of this chapter. Generally, these patients will also benefit from treatment for central pain disorder (Chapter 7).

POST-TRAUMATIC STRESS DISORDER

Tom was a fifty-six-year-old firefighter who came to my clinic. He was on disability and no longer working, and he presented with both severe neck pain and hip pain. His hip pain was found to be structural (severe hip arthritis), and we were able to adequately treat it with a hip replacement. However, his neck pain had not responded to conventional treatment. He had suffered for nine years with neck pain before seeing me and had tried several treatments, including neck epidural injections and a cervical spine surgery. None of this had worked. During our evaluation, he said, "I woke up from surgery in the same pain." He went on to get weekly massages and had eight sessions of acupuncture and two rounds of physical therapy. This gave him temporary relief but no real long-term progress.

I did an exam, which was remarkably normal except for some trigger points in his muscles. When I asked him when his symptoms would flare, he reported it was when he climbed stairs. That seemed like an unusual trigger. After diving deeper into his history, I discovered something that was not in any of the notes by his previous doctors. He was involved in a terrible fire ten years prior, where he was unable to rescue a child from the second floor of a home. The child ended up passing away, and my patient's brain took that guilt and emotional pain and converted it to neck pain. Each time he climbed a flight of stairs, his brain would subconsciously revisit that trauma, which elicited his pain.

Once we were able to identify the source, we worked through the MBPS program along with his psychologist, and he was able to make remarkable progress. He is now pain-free when he employs the techniques he learned.

Post-traumatic stress disorder (PTSD) occurs in people who have been exposed to or threatened by death, injury, or sexual violence. It greatly impacts one's life because sufferers of PTSD repeatedly relive the traumatic event and avoid trauma-related environments. As you can imagine, this triggers very high levels of cortisol and the activation of the fight-or-flight system. It is a severely challenging emotional state and is often treated with a combination of medications and psychotherapy.

PTSD has long been shown to be tied to the development of chronic pain. A group of researchers looked at 477 studies and found a significant link between PTSD and the subsequent development of chronic pain.[48]

A number of models have been proposed to explain how PTSD triggers physical pain.

1. The first is that the trauma triggers an arousal response that activates the sympathetic nervous system (SNS). With time, this overworked arousal system loses its ability to cope with pain.[49]

2. The second is titled the *shared vulnerability model* and proposes that patients with chronic pain and PTSD share a vulnerability to high levels of anxiety. As a result, their bodies have been primed, so when they do encounter an emotional stressor or a physical injury, their body has a heightened response and triggers pain.

3. The third model proposes that anxiety or SNS arousal is misinterpreted by the brain as pain. This is due to the body's inability to properly regulate stress hormones and biochemicals.[50]

Regardless of which theory is true, the treatment is still the same and will be covered in this chapter.

CONSEQUENCE OF BEING A HIGH-STRESS INDIVIDUAL

I find that quite a few patients with high levels of anxiety suffer from Mind-Body Pain Syndrome (MBPS). Some are unaware they even have anxiety because they have grown so accustomed to functioning at such high levels of fight-or-flight mode all the time.

Most of these people also do not have an official diagnosis of anxiety or depression despite manifesting signs of it. They just think being wound up and always "on" is part of their daily lives. Many are very successful and highly functioning individuals, such as financial advisors, attorneys, or CEOs of companies. Some are caregivers for sick family members; others are healthcare providers; and still others are essential workers in high-stress jobs, such as firemen and policemen. In many of these patients, there is no significant childhood or emotional/physical trauma that precipitated their pain. But by living at constant high levels of stress and anxiety, their autonomic nervous system is continuously in the "on" state.

Take John, for example. John was a twenty-four-year-old medical student that I saw while I was on faculty at the University of Chicago. He was a bright young man who had suddenly developed severe back pain during his first semester of school. He had an MRI of his back, which, due to his young age, was completely normal. He described occasional sciatica even though there was nothing on the MRI or physical exam to support this diagnosis. However, he described shooting, electrical pain down his leg and severe episodes of back pain that were disabling. Recently, the pain had gotten so severe that he was unable to go to his anatomy lab, and he was concerned he would not pass the class.

He also described symptoms of heartburn, tension headaches, and irritable bowel syndrome. He was on the rowing team in college, but due to this pain, he had stopped all physical activity. He did physical therapy as instructed by his primary doctor but reported it did not help him. After examining him and finding no evidence of a physical disorder to explain his pain, I told him I suspected his pain was from MBPS and fueled by his anxiety. I explained his pain was real but also curable. He started cognitive therapy, journaling, and doing daily meditation. In three weeks, he was ninety percent improved and back to exercising. After eight weeks, he had no pain.

As we have covered, chronic stress, such as that experienced by John, leads to increased sensitivity in your spinal cord, brain, and nerves. In John's case, I believe an overactive sympathetic nervous system was the precipitating factor, resulting in high levels of the hormone cortisol. Studies have shown adults with high levels of cortisol are more likely to develop chronic pain.[51] When your body is continuously in fight-or-flight mode, cortisol is secreted in excess, and we see a syndrome very similar to PTSD. In addition, chronic stress leads to a pro-inflammatory state.[52] But most importantly for John, an activated SNS triggered increased tension in his neck and back muscles, as well as activation of his GI tract.[53]

Another problem with remaining in this fight-or-flight state at all times is a number of negative lifestyle and physical factors occur (tightened shoulder and neck muscles, shallow breathing, poor exercise and sleep habits). All of these contribute to ongoing physical pain.

If this is you, I suggest working through this chapter as well as adopting a daily mindfulness and meditation practice. (See Chapter 14). The mindfulness practice is going to be key in handling future episodes of stress.

OTHER CAUSES OF MBPS

In some with MBPS, I have witnessed milder childhood traumas, current interpersonal conflicts, or feelings of guilt leading to pain syndromes. It takes a bit of digging to uncover these issues. I had one patient who felt her mother chose her job over her, another who felt they only received love from their father when they won a sports event, and another who, despite growing up to be an incredibly successful attorney, still experienced subconscious feelings of inadequacy related to when she was teased in middle school by classmates. As each of these patients identified and addressed their emotional triggers, they were able to pave a path to healing.

YOUR PAIN MAY BE WORSENED BY YOUR LABEL

Although labels can be helpful in identifying and treating disorders, as well as allowing other physicians to understand what's going on with a patient, I have found that the use of certain labels in certain ways can actually be damaging, as they can lead to stressors that can propagate ongoing pain. Consider the fact that in Norway *whiplash* as a diagnosis does not exist. Patients in Norway do not develop long-term pain issues after car accidents the same way we do. How is that possible?

A study done in Norway, a country where physicians recommend conservative management and immediate return to work after whiplash injuries, found that whiplash does not exist.[54,55] It found acute pain did happen, but chronic pain did not.

As we saw earlier, Mind-Body Pain Syndrome (MBPS) can be associated with a variety of symptoms involving multiple organ systems that are affected by your sympathetic nervous system. One can have fatigue, sleep disturbances, bowel symptoms, urinary symptoms, and pain. In our Western medical society, situations like this lead to someone having multiple diagnoses, seeing multiple specialists, getting dozens of tests, and being prescribed lots of medications. All of this can increase anxiety and further worsen their pain.[56]

Studies by White[57] indicated that the diagnostic label of fibromyalgia is in fact harmful to a patient because it creates this impression that there is a definite disease and pathology, but there is no cure. A Google search of "fibromyalgia treatment" alone will set almost anyone who recently received this diagnosis into a state of panic. This is because search results repeatedly claim there is no treatment or cure. The biochemical effect of this expectation itself may contribute to persistent pain and disability.

The reason goes back to the brain and one's expectation of injury, particularly one that is not reversible. The anxiety generated as a result of this type of diagnosis can perpetuate a chronic, incurable pain condition by being a continuous source of stress on your sympathetic nervous system.

YOUR DIAGNOSIS PERPETUATES INACTIVITY

Another consequence of having a "label" is many patients adopt maladaptive behaviors as a result. They feel that because they have a bad back or arthritis in the knee, they should decrease their activity levels to prevent further injury. This has clearly been shown to be detrimental because physical inactivity worsens muscle weaknesses that lead to imbalances, causing further pain.[58]

WHY HAVEN'T MY DOCTORS MENTIONED MBPS?

If medically reputable groups such as the IASP state that potential tissue damage, not just actual tissue damage, can cause pain, and the *DSM-V* has a diagnosis identifying Mind-Body Pain Syndromes, why is it that doctors who believe this system, like Dr. John Sarno, were seen as controversial? Why is it that Western doctors rarely bring up MBPS as a possible source for individuals with unexplained physical pain?

The answer is likely based on stigmas surrounding MBPS, the way conventional medicine is taught, and the cost benefit of more expensive treatments. However, as we continue to have skyrocketing healthcare costs related to chronic pain and are battling the opioid crisis with limited success, I am hopeful that the future will be different and more people will identify MBPS early in its course.

The next chapter will explain how to begin treating Mind-Body Pain Syndrome.

CHAPTER 6

MIND–BODY PAIN SYNDROME: RETRAIN YOUR PAIN BRAIN

"Pain is inevitable. Suffering is optional."
—Buddha

We learned the biology behind Mind-Body Pain Syndrome (MBPS) in the last chapter. This chapter will focus on how to treat it.

YOU CAN CONTROL YOUR PAIN BRAIN

In the last chapter we learned how our brain and revved-up nervous system can trigger physical pain symptoms. It is important to understand that although the pain is felt in the body, it can only be effectively treated by targeting your brain.

We have all heard examples of how our brain can overcome and control our physical symptoms. You may have read stories of mothers entering burning buildings to save their children and not experiencing pain. Or seen professional athletes continue to play without displaying signs of physical pain, despite a game-time injury. These individuals' brains have chosen not to experience pain at that time.

One study describes researchers asking twenty-nine female subjects to endure pain on behalf of their partners. They found through fMRI studies and follow-up questioning that their response to pain was decreased by doing this "favor" for their loved ones.[1]

Another study showed that displaying positive images and using guided imagery techniques trigger parts of the brain that lower pain levels.[2]

As you may recall from the last chapter, researchers have identified through fMRI studies that parts of the brain control the ability to modify how your body interprets pain signals. They have also found that this pathway can be altered to express less pain through positive social interactions and thoughts.

When individuals associate pain with something that has a positive consequence for others, such as volunteering or subjecting oneself to pain for the benefit of a loved one, the brain shifts so that it doesn't process the pain as painful.[3,4]

SUCCESSFULLY TREATING MIND-BODY PAIN SYNDROME

The key component to treating MBPS is making the diagnosis, accepting it, and intervening with thought restructuring and stress management. If we are able to do this early, we can break the pain cycle before central sensitization takes place.

Unfortunately, this is rarely done, as most doctors are trained to attribute pain to a physical cause. Even more unfortunately, through this process, they give the patient a number of diagnoses that only exacerbate their anxiety levels.

In his work, Dr. Sarno describes dozens of patients whose pain melted away as soon as they realized that nothing was physically wrong with them and that their emotions were triggering their pain. Their pain was so strongly tied to a fear of something being structurally wrong that as soon as they realized it was actually their mind creating the pain, the pain disappeared.

This may sound too good to be true, or at least too good to be that simple. And in many cases, especially those with severe trauma, it is. Although simply knowing that they had power over their pain through their minds has helped a handful of my patients, many required a lot more work. Luckily, we have been able to successfully treat them using the techniques listed below.

For those who have suffered severe trauma, I am truly sorry. Working through those experiences is often incredibly difficult to do on your own, and you may need the help of a trained and understanding professional. If, at any point, these exercises become too overwhelming, stop and seek help. The type of damage MBPS has caused your body is often so deeply ingrained that it takes months and specialized techniques to heal. Please do not hesitate to utilize both individual and group therapy, as well as the providers I recommend throughout this chapter. I encourage you to use this workbook with your counselor.

Remember, you are already beginning your healing process by reading this chapter and understanding that your brain controls your physical pain. Our next step is to break the cycle.

I recommend the following four approaches to treatment that we will address in this book.

1. CBT (THOUGHT RESTRUCTURING)

Dr. Sarno believed a key component to a patient's success was deconstructing their belief that their pain was a permanent condition, and empowering them with ways to tackle their internal emotional conflicts.

Lending additional support to this idea, a large number of scientific studies have been done on the treatment of somatoform disorders. As you may recall, somatoform disorders were described in the last chapter as severe forms of mind–body syndromes that are well understood in Western medicine. The most promising treatment studied so far for somatoform disorders is cognitive behavioral therapy or CBT.[5] CBT is a subset of psychotherapy that focuses on changing patterns of behavior and thinking to eventually change how someone feels and interprets situations. It focuses on the stress and anxious thoughts that are causing the physical symptoms. They have found CBT not only reduces the frequency and intensity of pain episodes, but also improves function and saves money on healthcare.[6,7,8]

As we dive into the exercises in this chapter, we will be doing a home-based modified CBT-type program that will allow you to identify and resolve emotional conflicts and stressors.

2. SELF-AFFIRMATION

How we perceive ourselves is something that is established very early in life and often related to our caregivers and how we were raised. Claude Steele is a psychologist who described the self-affirmation theory in the late 1980s. It refers to your self-worth and how you perceive yourself. The theory is that people inherently want to be perceived as good.

The self-affirmation theory goes even further to say people actually strive for self-integrity on a more global level. For example, if you donate your time and volunteer for an organization you believe in, this would lead to positive feelings that you are an inherently good person. Or if your parents, whose opinion you really value, tell you how proud they are of the person you have become. The positive feelings of self-worth that result from this one activity would in turn lead to positive feelings in other parts of your life.

An important aspect of self-affirmation is that maintaining this global "goodness" leads to positive outcomes in other aspects of one's life. For example, if someone feels good about themselves in one area, they are better able to tolerate a threat to their self-integrity in another area. This is a key factor in our body's resilience and response to stress. Those that have a higher sense of self-worth are more likely to tolerate negative events that take place.

Self-affirmation has been shown to increase activity in reward-related regions of the brain that also reduce pain, such as the ventral striatum and ventromedial prefrontal cortex (VMPFC).[9]

Self-affirmation is an important tool in recovering from Mind-Body Pain Syndrome. We will work through some exercises to incorporate this into your daily life.

3. MEDITATION AND MINDFULNESS PRACTICE

This will be covered in greater detail in Chapter 14. Please refer to that chapter.

4. MOVEMENT

MBPS needs to be treated with exercise or physical therapy as much as thought restructuring.

Sometimes, finding a way to resolve internal conflicts and remove external stressors calms one's nervous system, and many people's muscle pain eases up quite quickly. These individuals typically do not need focused physical therapy but do benefit from whole-body exercise programs that incorporate a mindfulness aspect. By adding meditation and deep breathing to movement, in practices such as yoga and tai chi, you promote relaxation of your sympathetic nervous system. This type of exercise favorably alters your stress hormones and leads to further reduction in your pain. I highly recommend incorporating these two to three times per week.

SUMMARY

Before we dive into the treatment worksheets, I want to summarize the general takeaway points, because we covered a lot of science in this chapter and the last. I feel there are two general subsets of individuals that develop MBPS.

1. Those that are chronically stressed and always anxious about day-to-day situations (big job interview, financial concerns, interpersonal relationships, whether their kids will get to school on time, etc.).

2. Those that have suffered an emotional trauma, abuse, PTSD, or have an ongoing internal conflict that has not yet been addressed or resolved (unhappy marriage, conflicts with parents, etc.).

Like our pain syndromes, these two groups often overlap.

TAKEAWAY POINTS

WHY WE GET MIND-BODY PAIN SYNDROME

Those who have experienced previous traumas, as well as those who haven't but who live under continuous heightened levels of stress, are primed for developing MBPS. This is due to the fact that an extended period of sympathetic nervous system activity (the fight-or-flight response) triggers pain pathways in the brain, impacting the brain's resilience to stress.

WHY UNRESOLVED EMOTIONAL CONFLICTS LEAD TO MBPS

1. Imaging studies have confirmed that the activity of pain pathways is altered by stress, positive emotions, and negative emotions. These are unrelated to a physical pain stimulus.

2. If your system has suffered a major trauma, either as a child or adult, these unresolved feelings of hurt and suffering lead to continuous stress on your sympathetic nervous system. This hormone imbalance causes you to enter into a pain cycle.

3. If you are continuously functioning at high levels of stress, or fight-or-flight mode, you will suffer similar negative chemical effects as those in #2.

4. Once your body has been primed by #2 or #3, any type of stressful event or state of anxiety can turn on your pain cycle, because your pathways are already primed to develop chronic pain.

5. As long as your unresolved conflicts exist or you continue to remain perpetually anxious, you will continue to fuel your nervous system to remain stuck in a pain cycle.

6. Scientists believe if you suffered childhood emotional trauma or PTSD, central sensitization has taken place. Please refer to the therapies suggested in Chapter 7 as well.

7. The key to healing is acceptance that the physical pain is your brain's expression of the trauma or unresolved conflict you experienced (or are currently experiencing). Once you have accepted this, you need to work to remove those emotional triggers.

8. In addition to the therapies illustrated in this book, you are likely to benefit from professional counseling and neurofeedback (see Resources section). For those suffering from PTSD, I highly suggest reading *The Body Keeps the Score* by Dr. Bessel van der Kolk.

WHY STRESS LEADS TO PAIN AND HOW TO BREAK THE CYCLE

1. When we are stressed, our sympathetic nervous system (SNS) is activated, and we contract our muscles, hunch forward, and tighten our necks. Studies have shown that when we are anxious or angry, we increase tension in our back.

2. Our fear of the diagnosis, and fear that we will never recover, adds additional fuel to the sympathetic nervous system fire, and the cycle of stress continues.

3. These changes are temporary. The tension you have is causing muscle tension, nerve firing, and brain activity that is generating pain. But remember, this is temporary and reversible. You do not have permanent tissue damage, and you are going to recover.

4. Inactivity hurts us. Activity can heal you. Often, people in pain and also people that are anxious after being given a new diagnosis, such as herniated disc, are afraid to move. This inactivity leads to disuse syndrome, which has been proven to worsen pain. This is why outside of a few rare diagnoses, doctors rarely prescribe bed rest anymore in the setting of back pain.

5. If you suffer from MBPS, you need to accept the pain is not physical or structural. It is still real, but must be handled in a different way than pain that is physical or structural. Your brain is driving your pain cycle.

LET'S START TO HEAL

Note: If you are already in counseling or plan to seek counseling, you can use these sheets while working with your therapist.

THREE-WEEK WRITING PROGRAM FOR SELF-HEALING

This writing program aims to reduce the impact pain has on your daily life, teach you skills to cope better with pain, and improve your overall functioning.

You need to be aware that this process is going to work to uncover any repressed emotions and stressors that contribute to your pain. For some of you who suffered childhood traumas, it is possible you have suppressed those memories and emotions instead of dealing with them. The result is your body has created this pain syndrome to express your emotional pain. We are going to work to identify these emotions, so you can break your cycle and feel relief. For some, this will be a highly emotional process. Do not give up. If you need to take a break for a few days, take it. But return to the exercises. If you are able, I highly recommend you do these with a licensed professional.

The following pages are a workbook. I suggest you buy a spiral notebook or staple some sheets of paper together and work through this as if this is your homework. You can also print our companion guide (see Free Gift at the beginning of the book) and use that to work through these exercises.

This process will take three weeks and require you to do daily work.

For this to work, you need to realize that the pain you feel is emotional tension. You are going to learn to let that go.

I want you to repeat the following phrase three times: **"I deserve to be pain-free."**

STEP 1: ACCEPTANCE.

The single most important aspect to healing is acceptance. You do have pain. But you must accept that there is nothing *structurally* wrong with you. You have no broken bones, you do not have a bad back, and there is nothing that needs to be surgically repaired. A doctor is not going to be able to give you a pill or perform a surgery that will cure you. In fact, these things may make you worse by creating real damage to tissues or nerves.

But *you* can heal yourself.

STEP 2: GOAL SETTING

Answer the following questions in your notebook.

1. What are your goals for therapy? Try to be specific. For example, be a better father or be able to jog a mile again.

2. Try to write down three to five goals.

3. Every week, write down if you have some improvement, moderate improvement, or a lot of improvement toward reaching these goals.

THE DIAPHRAGMATIC BREATH

Many people think they simply do not have time in their day to meditate. The health benefits of relaxation are so profound that even five minutes of relaxation and effective breathing can lead to increased energy, less pain, and lower your fight-or-flight response so effectively that you are actually more effective when you return to work.

I like this breathing exercise because so many of us are shallow breathers all day long, and this is an easy change to implement with profound effects.

1. Start by sitting in a chair.

2. Place one hand on your belly and one hand on your chest. Take a normal breath and notice which hand moves more. This is how you normally breathe. For most, it will be your chest. This indicates you are shallow breathing.

3. Now take a deep breath until the hand on your belly moves out. That is how you should be breathing.

USING THE BREATH TO HEAL

1. Sit in a chair with your feet flat on the floor.

2. Take a deep, slow breath while counting to three in your head—hold it for four seconds—and then slowly let it go over a six-second count. Similar to your exhalation, we are going to start letting go of our pain.

3. For your next breath, close your eyes and shift your attention to how deep your breath is. Try to breathe in all the way from your abdomen.

4. For the next breath, allow yourself to be aware of your pain. Focus on what area hurts. It may change as you breathe. Pay attention to that.

5. For the next breath, pay attention to any emotional pain you may have: sadness, anxiety, guilt, or depression.

6. Imagine now that as you breathe out, you can let go of some of that pain. Now with your next breath, try to find it again. Focus on what that feels like, and breathe it out.

7. And finally, while continuing the slow deep breathing, focus your attention on a happy time in your life. Perhaps it is hugging your children, cuddling with a significant other, or eating your favorite meal. Take yourself to that scene and feel yourself in that moment. Focus on all the sensation you have in that scene: how you feel, how it tastes, what you smell.

ANOTHER FORM OF BREATHING

Another form of relaxation breathing is Dr. Andrew Weil's 4–7–8 breathing technique. For this, you will inhale through your nose to a count of four inside your head. Then hold your breath for seven. Finally, exhale completely through your mouth to a count of eight.

Do one of these two breathing exercises daily and ideally every two to three hours throughout the day. Record your pain score before and after the exercise. After you do the deep breathing, think about how you feel. Are you more relaxed? Are your thoughts any different?

Breathing can be an incredibly useful tool to help you relax, reset your mind, and refocus your thoughts.[10]

As you continue to truly master your breathing and relax, your pain should drop even further. If you are having trouble, you can do a guided meditation with an app such as Headspace (see Resources).

PROGRESSIVE MUSCLE RELAXATION

As we discussed earlier in the chapter, when we tighten our muscles, we are causing tension that leads to pain. This exercise will involve going through different groups of muscles, tensing them first for a few seconds, and then gradually releasing the tension. I want you to do this each day after you are done working through the written exercises.

1. Sit in a chair, with good posture, hands on lap. Wear loose, comfortable clothes.

2. Begin by practicing your deep breathing. You will continue this throughout the exercise.

3. Forehead

   a. Raise your eyebrows, tensing the forehead muscles, and hold for four seconds.

   b. After counting to four, take a deep breath in. Pause for two counts.

   c. As you exhale slowly, release the tension.

4. Face

   a. Clench your teeth together, wrinkle your nose, and tightly squeeze your eyes shut. Try to tense all the muscles in your face.

   b. Remain like this for a count of four.

   c. Take a deep breath in, hold for two counts, then exhale slowly and release the tension.

5. Neck/Shoulders

   a. Draw your shoulder blades back together.

b. Hold for four seconds. After, take a deep breath in, hold for two counts.

c. Then exhale slowly, releasing the tension.

6. Arms

a. Make a tight fist, bend your arm at your elbow, and bring it toward your shoulder.

b. Feel the tension in your arms and hold for four seconds.

c. Then take a deep breath in, hold for two seconds, then exhale slowly, releasing the tension.

7. Legs

a. Extend your leg out straight and tense your thighs. Hold for four seconds.

b. Then take a deep breath in and hold for two seconds. As you exhale slowly, release the tension.

8. Feet

a. Flex your foot by pulling your toes up. Feel the tension in your feet. Hold for four seconds.

b. Take a deep breath in. Hold for two seconds. As you exhale slowly, release the tension.

As you grow more accustomed to this practice, you will learn to do a whole-body muscle relaxation sequence on your own. Starting from your forehead, moving down your face, to shoulders, arms, hips, legs, ankles. End by deep breathing for one minute. You should do this at least once a day for the duration of the exercises in this chapter. If you find it is helping, continue to use this exercise daily.

WRITTEN EXERCISE #1: COGNITIVE RESTRUCTURING

I want you to make a list of four stressful events that took place in the last week that seemed to be tied to your pain, along with your thoughts at the time and reaction. If you can't think of any that specifically tie to your pain, think of any stressful events. You may later remember that you had pain at the time of this stressful event. Try to think of what that was. I will include an example below.

Stressful Event	Beliefs/Thoughts	Your Reaction
The traffic is so bad today! I'm going to be late to work again.	Why does this always happen to me? Will I get fired? Why can't I do anything right?	**Emotional** – Frustrated, angry, upset
		Physical – Headache, low back pain

We are now going to take steps to learn to restructure our thoughts.

1. Think back to your stressful situation.

2. Separate the thoughts into ones specifically related to the situation (What is my boss going to think?) and others that are more generally related to you (Why can't I do anything right?).

3. Look for which thoughts could be true in that given situation and what may not be true. I want you to then focus on replacing those negative thoughts with better positive thoughts. Write these down. First the negative thought and then an arrow to the replacement positive thought.

4. "I always get stuck in traffic." TO "I do often get stuck in traffic, but most of the time the traffic lightens up and I get to work on time. I have only been late to work once in the last

three months. My boss will understand if I am five minutes late. Tomorrow I will leave even earlier."

5. "I can't do anything right." TO "The traffic jam is out of my control. I have gone through things much worse than a little traffic jam. My back hurts, but I'm learning ways to reduce my pain. I am going to get better."

6. It is important you begin to recognize every time you are in a stressful situation and the accompanying negative thoughts. You will need to develop your own positive mantras to say in those situations. Come up with three positive thoughts. Write these down in your journal.

WRITTEN EXERCISE #2: IDENTIFY PAST STRESSORS

CHILDHOOD

I want you to start by looking at your childhood caregivers and jotting down notes about your experiences, first with your mother and father. If you were raised by grandparents, uncles/aunts, just add them as needed. Be sure to note if there was any abuse in the house (sexual, emotional, or physical abuse) or any excessive substance use in any of your caregivers. Try to answer each of the following questions one by one.

1. Father: Describe your relationship: loving, warm, cold? Write words to describe him. How did he treat you? Any abuse? Any judgment? Any yelling? Did you feel loved?

2. Mother: How was your relationship: loving, warm, cold? Write words to describe her. How did she treat you? Any abuse? Any judgment? Any yelling? Did you feel loved?

3. How was your parents' relationship? Did you see love? Did you witness any fighting or abuse?

4. Siblings: Did you have a good relationship with them? Any resentment? Did your parents treat you differently than them?

5. Friends: How was your relationship with your friends? Do any particularly negative events stand out? Were you bullied? Did you do any bullying?

6. Were you ever the victim of any unwanted sexual abuse or activity?

7. Did you ever feel not good enough or criticized? Who criticized you?

8. Were there any adults (teachers, coaches, etc.) that left negative experiences in your memory?

9. Was there any specific negative event that left an imprint in childhood? How about during your teenage or young adulthood years?

WRITTEN EXERCISE #3: TYING PAST STRESSORS TO PHYSICAL SYMPTOMS

Next, we are going to write out a timeline. This is very important in uncovering the chronology of your chronic pain and specific events that may be tied to it. You can do this by your age or year the event took place, whatever is easiest.

I want you to write down a list of all your symptoms and diagnoses related to your pain. Next to each item, I want you to write the dates you began to experience those symptoms. I want you also to note any important events (e.g., divorce, new job, death in family) that happened shortly before or at the time your various pain symptoms started. Try to dig deep into what past events or stressors may have been happening around the time of each symptom/disease onset.

Now I want you to evaluate your current relationships. Make a list of all the important relationships you currently have: family, close friends, work relationships, etc. Are any current relationships similar to any negative childhood relationships? For example, does your boss remind you of your overly critical father?

Remember, emotional pain builds over time. And each emotional injury is additional fuel for your fire. It is important to identify if there are any present relationships or situations that are similar to painful earlier memories. These can trigger our subconscious mind to relive all those earlier emotional issues and present as physical symptoms.

WRITTEN EXERCISE #4: IDENTIFY NEGATIVE FEELINGS

I want you to list the following in your journal:

1.   What things make you scared?

2.   What things make you angry?

3.   What things cause you to be resentful or jealous?

4.   What things give you either conscious or subconscious guilt?

What situations led you to experience these feelings? Give examples.

Once you know what led to them, you need to realize every experience has taught you something. What was that lesson? Now that you know the lesson, what action will you take so that it does not happen again?

EXPRESSIVE WRITING TO HELP HEAL CHRONIC PAIN

Once those structured writing assignments are complete, we will move into some additional writing exercises to work through your MBPS. These are less structured. The key to this type of expressive writing is that it is unstructured, free prose. Choose whatever writing method you are most comfortable with. For most people, this is writing by hand, but some prefer to type. I recommend not doing it on your phone, as it takes time to type on the notepad on your phone, and we want this writing to be free and fast. The writing is a way for your body to release your suppressed emotions that are manifesting as pain. Even if you are scribbling and it is mostly illegible, continue anyway.

To be effective, you must complete all the exercises, and be honest and detailed in your writing.

Each day, at the end of each writing exercise, I want you to write the following self-affirmation:

I am working toward eliminating my pain.
I am relieved to finally uncover the source of my pain.
I deserve to be happy.

WRITTEN EXERCISE #5: DETERMINING STRESSORS

Today we are going to identify all stressors and maladaptive feelings. I want you to write for fifteen to thirty minutes about all your current stressors in the last year. These may be work, family, finances, overcommitment, upcoming events such as weddings etc. Try to make this list as long and inclusive as possible.

WRITTEN EXERCISE #6: PAST STRESSORS OR TRAUMAS

Make a list of your past difficult experiences. These may be traumas, abuse, relationships that may have failed, friendships that ended, loss of a job, divorce, bullying, deaths in the family, etc.

We are digging now for priming events that may be the original source of your MBPS. (Whereas the current stressors from Day 5 are symptom-triggering events.)

This is the most important list you will create, because past experiences are the leading cause of MBPS. Some may seem trivial years later, like missing a soccer goal in a game, but they may have been very important at that time. It is also important to remember that the cumulative impact of past stressors is important to identify, so we must list any and all possible past stressful and traumatic events. Each one may seem minor, but when looked at as cumulative insults to your body, they become significant.

After each event, I want you to list how it made you feel (scared, angry, hurt, isolated, etc.). You can even discuss these with your parents and siblings, who may remember some traumatic experiences from your early childhood better than you do.

Try to write them in chronological order.

WRITTEN EXERCISE #7: IDENTIFY ASPECTS OF YOUR PERSONALITY THAT MAY BE DETRIMENTAL

Try to dig deep and take a look at yourself. Are you a type A perfectionist? Do you express emotions easily or bottle them up? Do you have difficulty saying no? Do you obsess over thoughts? Are you constantly worrying?

It is important to realize these are not negative qualities. In fact, some are seen as highly positive qualities and have probably led you to achieve success in your career, stand up for yourself, or be a great friend. But we are looking for things that may be causing repressed emotions in yourself that are manifesting as pain.

WRITTEN EXERCISE #8: SELF-CRITICISM

What do you think about yourself? Are you proud of all you have accomplished? Are you your worst critic?

Make a list of things you like about yourself and things you do not.

Now look at the things you do not like and break them down further. Use examples in your life of where those negative things have actually not been negative. For example, "I am not as good as Aria at my job." And replace with, "Aria has been doing this longer than me, so she does have more experience. However, I am doing a really good job at being organized, I received a lot of compliments from my boss on my last assignment, and compared to the others who started the same time as me, I am definitely just as good if not better."

It may be hard to write about the topics under Days 7-8 because it does require quite a bit of introspection, so if you are unable to identify them, I encourage you to just write about yourself and your feelings on a given day and then go back later and try to identify anything that may fall into a negative category. From there, try to reframe those thoughts.

For many, uncovering these stressors and negative thoughts may take several months of daily journaling or even working with a counselor or therapist.

WRITTEN EXERCISE #9: INTERPERSONAL RELATIONSHIPS

Today I want you to write for fifteen to twenty minutes about what others think about you and how that makes you feel. You can write about what your parents think/thought about you either now or in the past, what you have been told about yourself by your boss or family, and how that made you feel. What are your favorite relationships right now? Least favorite?

WRITTEN EXERCISE #10: ACCOMPLISHMENTS AND FAILURES

Reflect on your whole life and write for fifteen to twenty minutes. Create one list of things you are proud of and another list of things you are ashamed of. Include both past and recent experiences. Separate these lists into two columns.

For the list of events you are ashamed of, go back to your timeline and see if it correlates with the onset or worsening of any of your symptoms. If you find that it does, write the following down.

"_____ event triggered my pain. There is nothing physically wrong with me. Now that I have identified the cause, and I accept the event is over, my life can move on, and I can let go of the pain."

I want you to write this down five times or repeat it out loud five times each day, followed by the progressive muscle relaxation exercise. Do this for ten days.

This same exercise can be done for any of the events or relationships through these exercises that you discover may have triggered your pain.

WRITTEN EXERCISE #11: CONTRIBUTING EVENT

I want you to pick the stressor or event that you feel has contributed the most to your pain. What past negative experiences or thoughts keep creeping into your mind? What have you missed out on as a result of these negative thoughts? I want you to write for ten minutes about that experience and be very specific. Do not stop.

After the ten minutes, I want you to write for another ten minutes about three ways you can challenge your negative thoughts.

For the last five minutes, I want you to write about how you can change when these thoughts come up again. Refer to the cognitive restructuring exercise from earlier.

DO THIS FOR ANOTHER EVENT AS WRITTEN EXERCISE #12.

WRITTEN EXERCISE #13: FEARS

I want you to answer the following questions. What things am I afraid of? How are those fears holding me back? Write for fifteen to twenty minutes.

WRITTEN EXERCISE #14: REFLECT

Today I want you to write for fifteen to twenty-five minutes as a self-reflection on what these exercises have taught you about yourself. Be sure to compliment yourself on all the hard work you have done!

If you have found this helpful, I want you to continue to set aside ten to fifteen minutes a day to journal your feelings and experiences.

I want you to get in the habit, as you write, of feeling like you are healing. By processing your thoughts, you are releasing them from your body and therefore releasing all that pent-up physical pain that is caused by repressed emotions and anxiety.

Remember to always use positive self-affirmation in your thoughts throughout the day and at the end of your journaling/meditation. You can create your own or use the ones we mentioned in this chapter.

LETTER WRITING

We are now going to begin writing letters to heal and release these emotions we have uncovered in the first two weeks of our exercises. You do not have to *send* the letter, though you may want to consider sending these letters, as it is possible some people who have deeply hurt you are unaware of the harm they have caused you. It is possible that by opening up to them and having this discussion, you can begin to truly heal. Even if you do not reach a resolution with that individual, telling them how you feel can be part of the healing process.

I want you to write four letters. The letters will be described below. You can write this in one day or over four days. Again, just freely write your feelings without regard to punctuation or neatness. If you choose to share them with the individual(s), you can rewrite the letter, or type it up, at a later time.

Written Exercise #15: Letter #1. Write a letter to whomever you are angry at or have issues with. This could be a spouse, parent, child, or friend. You may need to write multiple letters. These may be people you are not ready to forgive. Write them a letter anyway.

Written Exercise #16: Letter #2. Write a letter to someone you are angry with but want to forgive. This can be a second letter to everyone you wrote to on Day 15.

Written Exercise #17: Letter #3. Write a letter to your parents. Include things you appreciate them for and things you may not have appreciated them for.

Written Exercise #18: Letter #4. Write a letter to yourself. If there is anything you are angry at or disappointed in yourself for, I want you to write a letter of forgiveness to yourself. I want you to be kind in this letter and recognize your positives. If there are things you are ashamed of, acknowledge and accept those things in writing in this letter. Always end with positive thoughts.

GRATITUDE: THE POWER OF POSITIVITY

We are going to end our writing exercises with gratitude journaling. This is something you should be doing regularly. Even if you do not write it down, after these exercises are complete, I want you to continue to express gratitude in your daily life. Gratitude has incredible healing powers.

Each day, think of three things you are grateful for. For these exercises, we will dive a little further.

WRITTEN EXERCISE #19: LETTER #5.

I want you to start by writing a letter to somebody who positively impacted your life. Write this letter to someone who helped you in some way, shape, or form.

WRITTEN EXERCISE #20: GRATITUDE LIST.

I want you to make a list of what you are grateful for. Answer the questions below:

1. Who in your life are you grateful for? Why?

2. What special skills or traits do you possess that you are grateful for?

3. What parts of your life are you grateful for?

4. What positive events have happened to you over the last ten years?

5. What foods are you most grateful for?

6. What aspects of your family are you grateful for?

7. What hobbies/interests are you grateful for that you can still do?

8. What part of nature gives you the most enjoyment?

9. What part of where you live brings you joy?

10. What people in your life bring you joy?

Try to incorporate fifteen minutes of gratitude journaling every week. You can follow the following format:

Date:

I am grateful for:

Reflection of thoughts:

You can also expand on this format and take it beyond words. You can fill your notebook up however you wish. Think of moments you are grateful for and place items in your journal to commemorate those memories, such as photos, movie ticket stubs, or collages. You can even buy positivity stickers for $5–$8 on Amazon or make up positive affirmation statements to write on the pages of your journal.

MOVING FORWARD: SCHEDULING IN SOME FUN

Too often, chronic pain leaves us depressed and withdrawn. Often, we give up on hobbies and activities we once enjoyed, either because we feel they will induce pain or we simply don't have the energy or motivation to do them.

That needs to change starting today! This exercise asks you to find a list of activities you enjoy that you can physically do. If there are activities you can do with friends or loved ones, even better! Social support and community are components of living well and pain-free.

I want you to list as many activities as you can that you enjoy and that are feasible to still participate in. They may include things like the following: have lunch with my friends, play a board game with my daughter, dance to my favorite song, write in my journal, read a book.

Then I want you to try to schedule two to three of them every week for the next two months. You can schedule them on a paper calendar or in your phone calendar, but make sure to actually schedule them in and do them!

MANAGING A PAIN CRISIS

Despite working through this chapter, you are still likely to have flares of your pain. It is important to know how to utilize the tools you have been taught in this book to handle the flares.

Learn to anticipate when a flare of pain may come based on recording your usual emotional triggers in a journal.

Start by reminding yourself there is nothing structurally wrong with you. Tell yourself your symptoms are indicating something else is going on and you need to find out what those triggers/causes are. Are you angry, scared, anxious, resentful, guilty? Take a deep breath, and tell yourself you can control those emotions and the pain will go away. If you need to, jot down a list of what is bothering you emotionally and remind your brain that you will address these emotions one by one so your brain does not need to trigger the pain.

Practice using restructured thinking and positive statements to reframe negative thoughts. Keep a list of affirmation statements in your notebook. Or write them on index cards or Post-its and place them on your bathroom mirror as a daily reminder.

Remember to do your diaphragmatic breathing and progressive muscle relaxation exercises when feeling anxious or experiencing pain. These can immediately reduce your fight-or-flight system activation. Every three to four hours, deep breathe for a minute.

When you make it through the flare, remember to add self-affirmations and positive thoughts about how well you managed it. You can write them down or say them to yourself. I want you to learn to encourage and compliment yourself.

Each day you will carve out time for ten minutes of meditation or progressive muscle relaxation. Try to keep a daily log.

ADDITIONAL THERAPY MODALITIES FOR MBPS

As I stated earlier in the chapter, movement is a huge component of healing Mind-Body Pain Syndrome (MBPS) and often is a vital adjunct to cognitive therapy. I suggest you take a peek at the physical pain chapters (Chapters 3 and 4) to assess for muscular imbalances. If you have some, I recommend you address them or get evaluated by a physical therapist.

Exercise has been shown to have profound effects on the stress response cycles, by balancing our hypothalamic pituitary adrenal (HPA) axis.[11]

I highly recommend exercise that incorporates a mind–body aspect. My preferred modalities for patients with MBPS are yoga, tai chi, Feldenkrais, or somatic movement. You should do these at least two to three times a week.

YOGA

Yoga is a spiritual exercise practice from India that combines breathing techniques, meditation, and exercise. See Resources for free online videos. Yoga has been shown to help with a variety of pain conditions, such as chronic low back pain and joint pain,[12] but if you are new to exercising you should start under the guidance of a physical therapist. You can even look for a physical therapist that is a certified yoga instructor as well if this interests you.

TAI CHI

Tai Chi is a low-impact mind–body exercise from China with slow, prescribed movements with attention to breathing and meditation. One hundred seven systematic reviews confirmed its potential benefit for chronic pain syndromes.[13,14] You can look to see if your nearby park center, YMCA, or senior center offers free or discounted classes. YouTube has some beginner tai chi videos available for free.

(Check out videos from Taiflow.) This is typically physically easier to do than yoga.

FELDENKRAIS

Feldenkrais is a method of mind–body awareness training, where you are guided through a series of movements that explore different senses. This can be done in a group or individual setting. The purpose of these explorations is to practice the process of sensing the difference between two or more options to achieve a stated movement, and subsequently choosing the option that allows you to do the movement with less effort and pain. These movements and thoughts are predicated on a judgment that is positive (pleasurable, easy, and with less effort) compared with an experience of exercise that may give you pain or discomfort. Further, the participants are encouraged to generate alternative movements that work for them. Feldenkrais can be done by patients who have limited activity levels.

In my opinion, self-directed Feldenkrais is challenging, so this modality may not be an easy one to transition to as a home program. You can go to the Feldenkrais website to learn more, watch a sample video, and find a local class or event (http://www.feldenkrais.com/). Classes generally cost about $10–$20, but packages may be available at certain locations.

SOMATIC MOVEMENT

Feldenkrais may be difficult to learn on your own, but luckily a similar type of practice exists. It is called *somatic movement*, and it also incorporates a mind–body awareness aspect. Patients typically find this one easier to master at home. You can visit this website (https://somaticmovementcenter.com/)to learn more. There is an online course for $45, as well as some free exercise videos on the website.

FINDING A PRACTITIONER

If you have not improved after our worksheets and starting an exercise program, I *strongly* suggest you find a practitioner trained specifically in Mind-Body Pain Syndrome. See Resources.

For those who can't, you should seek out a local biofeedback and cognitive behavioral therapy practitioner who specializes in chronic pain.

For those who can't afford either option, the Resources section has books, apps, and websites to help in your quest to eliminate Mind-Body Pain Syndrome.

BIOFEEDBACK

As we have seen, our revved-up sympathetic nervous systems cause pain. Biofeedback is a safe, non-invasive treatment that allows patients to learn to control physiological responses to pain.

In a biofeedback session, a patient is hooked up to monitors that allow the therapist and patient to measure physiological activities, such as breathing, heart rate, brain waves, muscle tension, and skin temperature. They then work through thoughts, resulting emotions, and physical responses to these varying stimuli. A surface electromyography (EMG) is placed to detect muscle tension, along with a skin temperature probe, an EEG monitor for brain waves, and a heart monitor to detect heart rate variability and rhythms.

The measurements are specifically targeted to those that would be hyperactive in states of sympathetic nervous system arousal, which is why it is particularly helpful in both Mind-Body Pain Syndrome and Central Pain Syndrome.

EMG biofeedback has been shown to be beneficial for stress and anxiety,[15] low back pain,[16] headaches,[17] and TMJ disorders.[18] Neurobiofeedback or EEG biofeedback has been shown effective for PTSD,[19] trigeminal neuralgia,[20] CRPS,[21] and fibromyalgia.[22]

You can find a therapist practicing biofeedback by searching the Biofeedback Certification International Alliance website at www.bcia.org. For research on biofeedback and an additional list of providers, please visit the Association for Applied Psychophysiology and Biofeedback at www.aapb.org.

AT-HOME OPTIONS

There are a handful of options to use at home, but I personally think they are hefty investments and the learning curve is quite steep, so it may not be worth it without professional guidance first.

Once you acquire biofeedback skills with a professional, there are some at-home neurobiofeedback systems that patients have success with—for example, emWave2 (HeartMath). These tend to be relatively easy to use and provide benefit, but I do not feel it is the same as going to an in-person session.

You should also be aware that there are a lot of devices out there that tout themselves as biofeedback devices, when they do not work. These devices are not regulated, so be sure to do your research before spending your money.

Another technique patients have found success from is emotional freedom tapping (EFT). For more information, you can refer to the Resources.

COGNITIVE BEHAVIORAL THERAPY

A therapist specifically using cognitive behavioral therapy (CBT) can also be extremely helpful. This therapy is an extension of what we did in this chapter and enables you to work on restructuring faulty thought processes to achieve pain relief.

As you transition to greater self-awareness, know that you are taking steps to improve your health and reduce your pain. This takes time, like anything in my program, because you need to unlearn faulty thought processes and reframe your brain chemistry. But with dedication and time, you will break through your pain cycle.

CHAPTER 7

CENTRAL PAIN SYNDROME: HEALING BRAIN AND BODY INFLAMMATION

"Although the world is full of suffering,
it is also full of the overcoming of it."
—Helen Keller

Noreen, a thirty-four-year-old female, presented to my clinic with migraine headaches, chronic neck pain, and irritable bowel syndrome. She had seen multiple specialists for her issues, including her primary care physician, a gastroenterologist, a neurologist, and a psychiatrist. She was diagnosed with myofascial pain and migraine headaches. Despite trying over eight different medications for depression and headaches, her migraines had not improved.

An integrative approach was utilized to treat Noreen's pain. Trigger point injections and cupping were used to treat her neck myofascial pain. An elimination diet identified gluten as a trigger for her migraines. Stool analysis identified bacterial overgrowth, which was treated with antibiotics, probiotics, and enzymes. Micronutrient deficiencies were identified and treated. She began an exercise and stress-reduction program at home. Within six months, she was no longer having migraines, neck pain, or GI symptoms and had weaned off all her medications.

WHAT IS CENTRAL PAIN SYNDROME?

Central Pain Syndrome (CPS) is the most challenging syndrome to treat of all three syndromes. CPS syndromes are typically found in individuals with one or more of the following conditions: autoimmune conditions, rheumatological diseases, fibromyalgia, chronic fatigue syndrome, migraine headaches, pelvic pain, irritable bowel syndrome, complex regional pain syndrome, inflammatory bowel syndrome, interstitial cystitis, or bladder pain.

It is very important that if you suffer from Central Pain Syndrome, you have seen a physician to rule out conditions that are treatable, such as vitamin D deficiency, hypothyroidism, cancer, and autoimmune conditions. If you have experienced significant amounts of unintentional weight gain or weight loss, I recommend seeing a medical doctor right away.

BIOLOGY BEHIND CENTRAL PAIN

REVVED-UP NERVOUS SYSTEM

Central Pain Syndrome is a disorder caused by nervous system inflammation. In other words, parts of your nervous system become hyperactive and enter into a cycle of constant inflammation.

This inflammation begins when our nervous systems are "turned on." Our nervous system houses glial cells, which are the glue that connects other cells of the brain. Microglia are the immune cells of the brain and are involved in processes critical for the maintenance of our nervous system. When these cells become persistently activated by an injury to either the peripheral or central nervous system, our brain's immune system can no longer work properly.

Some examples of peripheral injury include trauma, bacterial infections, viral infections, and environmental toxins.[1] Some central nervous system triggers are emotional trauma or severe stress.[2] Although you can sometimes have a single attributing cause trigger the onset of centralized pain, most of the time it evolves as a consequence of multiple assaults to the microglia.

This stimulation to this system, either by a single trigger or multiple assaults to our microglia, leads to a constant neuroinflammatory state. This state leads to hyperreactivity of the central nervous system. Neurons in your body become sensitized and hyperresponsive by way of an excitatory neurotransmitter chemical called *glutamate*. Glutamate activates the NMDA receptor, a receptor which plays a key role in the development of Central Pain Syndrome. The NMDA receptors, once activated, increase in number and lead to a rewiring of the brain. In short, the brain has now become more sensitive to pain.

Experts believe the increased excitability of nerve cells in the spinal cord results in the symptoms we see most often with central pain disorders. Think of it like being stuck in a room with music blasting at the highest volume, and the volume controller has been broken. In central sensitization, our nervous system has become so excited it can no longer amplify that noise. It is constantly "on" and revved up, leading to pain. This means that for those suffering from central pain, stimuli that used to be seemingly harmless now cause significant pain. This is known as *allodynia*. An example is someone who feels pain when they are lightly touched. Another common physical characteristic of central pain we see is *hyperalgesia*: pain levels experienced are much higher than we would expect. In people suffering from central pain, even a hug or a cool summer breeze can be painful.

Pain receptors that can be overly sensitized are found in muscle, fascia, and other areas of the body. In addition to a heightened sensation of pain, all this hyperexcitation causes our brains to suffer, and Central Pain Syndrome promotes depression, anxiety, and fatigue. It can even lead to loss of gray matter volume in the brain, similar to a neurodegenerative disease such as Alzheimer's dementia.[3]

ABNORMAL MITOCHONDRIA

Mitochondria are key players in our body. They are the energy factory for all of our cells and are in charge of running all cellular activities. Their most important function is that of aerobic respiration, which is the process by which food is converted to energy using oxygen. They are also in charge of shutting down the energy factory when enemies are encountered, such as infections, inflammation, and toxins. When this happens, they switch roles and work to defend cells. If the outside attack is very strong, the mitochondria can actually die, leading to suboptimal function of whatever organ they are in.

In summary, your mitochondria control your ability to fight foreign invaders, your response to stressors, your energy level, and your overall body function.

Central Pain Syndrome can be triggered by mitochondrial dysfunction. It has been shown that patients with fibromyalgia and complex regional pain syndrome (CRPS), our most commonly studied Central Pain Syndromes, demonstrate abnormal mitochondrial function. They have found lower numbers of mitochondria in these patients, and those mitochondria that are present are destroyed and smaller in size.[4,5]

MITOCHONDRIAL MALFUNCTION = OXIDATIVE STRESS = WIDESPREAD MUSCLE PAIN

It is not uncommon for patients suffering from Central Pain Syndromes, like fibromyalgia, to have chronic widespread muscle pain. They have found these patients have increased levels of glutamate and lactate in their muscles—a sign of impaired mitochondrial function.[6] Fascia, the strong stretchy tissue on top of the muscles, is also a common source of pain for patients with fibromyalgia and other Central Pain Syndromes.

POSSIBLE CAUSES OF CENTRAL PAIN SYNDROMES

I will begin this section by introducing some conditions leading to Central Pain Syndrome (CPS) that can be treated. Please work with your healthcare practitioner to rule these out first, and then move on to the treatment plan. If you suffer from CPS, you will likely require blood work and possible advanced lab testing to rule out these causes.

INFECTIONS

Sometimes certain infections can cause long-term problems with our immune systems.[7] It is postulated that these infectious particles attach to glial cells and cause the central nervous system hyperactivity we described earlier. A functional medicine practitioner or primary care doctor can help investigate these as possible causes.

Many functional medicine (FM) practitioners believe candida (yeast) overgrowth can cause fibromyalgia and other Central Pain Syndromes. However, to date, there has not been an overwhelming amount of evidence to support that notion. Despite this lack of evidence, FM practitioners have reported large numbers of fibromyalgia patients having yeast (candida) infections due to recurrent antibiotic use. Once treated, these patients experienced improvement of fibromyalgia symptoms. However, these results have not yet been proven in clinical trials. If you do suspect you have yeast overgrowth, or have a history of long-term antibiotic use, you can discuss this with your doctor.

Various viruses have been studied as triggering pain conditions such as fibromyalgia, neuropathy (nerve pain), irritable bowel syndrome, and rheumatoid arthritis.[8] Scientists at Stanford have been studying chronic fatigue syndrome and found links indicating that it may result from either a viral or bacterial infection. Dr. John Chia, an infectious disease doctor, has reported a number of findings suggesting an association of chronic fatigue syndrome (CFS) with enteroviruses. Enteroviruses are very common infections that routinely give us mild symptoms of cough, runny nose, gastrointestinal (GI) symptoms, and body aches. Dr. Chia observed that patients with chronic fatigue commonly have GI complaints, and a large number have irritable bowel syndrome.[9] His group found a protein marker of enterovirus in eighty-two percent of stomach biopsy samples of CFS patients. In many patients, the initial viral infection was years ago, but the virus had triggered their CFS, and the persistent infection continued to cause symptoms.[10]

Reports are now appearing about COVID-19 causing a post-viral pain syndrome and chronic fatigue symptoms. I have a few patients who suffered the infection who are reporting these symptoms months later. Although we are still investigating effective treatments for COVID-19, the principles in this chapter, as well as Part 2, will be helpful in improving these symptoms once the virus has passed.

Some chronic infections that can be treated include vaginitis, sinusitis, or dental infections. Other infections that should be explored as etiologies include Lyme disease, Epstein-Barr virus (mononucleosis), parasites, hepatitis A, B, or C, HIV, mycoplasma infections, and chlamydia.

Diagnosis of underlying infections is key because if the infectious trigger is identified, you may find relief with appropriate antimicrobial therapy (antivirals, antifungals, or antibiotics).

IRON OVERLOAD

Genetic hemochromatosis (iron overload) can cause persistent muscle pain (tested by the blood test ferritin). Iron deficiency should also be ruled out via a ferritin blood test. This can be easily ordered by your primary doctor.

AVENUES OF TREATMENT

To date, central sensitization is poorly understood and subsequently poorly treated. Doctors primarily utilize medications to treat symptoms, such as antidepressants or opioids. These do not effectively treat the underlying cause and thus have limited benefit. Others may receive no treatment and are told it is in their head. Fibromyalgia is not simply a diagnosis of psychogenic origin (i.e., it is a real disease and not just in your head). However, the mental aspect is still a key component of treatment. As we saw above, stress is a common trigger for peripheral inflammation, leading to brain inflammation. In fact, if this was the only trigger, once addressed and treated appropriately (see Chapter 5), patients can have significant improvement in symptoms.

Many people with fibromyalgia and other Central Pain Syndromes respond favorably to additional therapies described in this chapter that conventional medicine rarely explores.

The first step in achieving relief from central pain is understanding which components contribute to this pain cycle. Nervous system inflammation and mitochondrial dysfunction are the two root causes of Central Pain Syndromes. Therefore both must be treated to obtain relief. When it comes to Central Pain Syndromes, conventional medicine tends to focus solely on masking symptoms and rarely addresses these issues.

ROLE OF THE IMMUNE SYSTEM IN CENTRAL PAIN

As stated above, complex regional pain syndrome and fibromyalgia are the most studied central sensitization syndromes. Both of these commonly have allodynia (feeling pain from something that should not cause pain, such as a breeze) and hyperalgesia (heightened sensation of pain) as presenting signs. Both have also been shown to have immune system triggers tied to the disease onset.[11] In short, a revved-up immune system leads to these issues.

We have seen plenty of pro-inflammatory states, the most common being obesity. Obesity is a proinflammatory state. Because of this, it is important that nutrition and weight be addressed in the treatment of central pain.

Many studies have shown a link between fibromyalgia and obesity. Obesity impacts our body's ability to regulate pain via the hypothalamic-pituitary-adrenal (HPA) axis (our hormone control center) and also leads to elevated levels of inflammation, which could be driving this disease for some individuals.

An important contributor to our levels of inflammation and overall increasing chronic disease is diet and obesity. Please refer to Chapter 10 for recommendations on an anti-inflammatory/anti-pain diet.

IS IT AUTOIMMUNE?

One thing to keep in mind if you have signs of centralized pain is that you may suffer from an early autoimmune disorder that has not yet been diagnosed.

See the table below and circle all the symptoms you have.

Acid reflux/GERD	Asthma	Digestive issues	Hair loss
ADHD	Eczema	Dry eyes	Weight gain/loss
Seasonal allergies	Vitamin deficiencies	Kidney disease	Headaches
Food allergies	Brain fog	Fatigue	Infertility
Anxiety	Type 2 diabetes	Rashes	Sleep issues
Pancreatitis	Depression	Gallstones	Swollen joints

If you suffer from eight to ten of the above conditions, in addition to pain, keep in mind that you may have an autoimmune condition. If you suffer from even three to four of them, you likely have a low level of underlying inflammation that should be addressed from a dietary standpoint (see Chapter 10).

I suggest you see your primary care doctor or a rheumatologist first to get some baseline lab work. (In doctor speak, those labs would include CBC, BMP, CRP, ESR, TSH, Vit D [serum 25(OH)D], ferritin, Mg, Vit B_{12}, ANA, CCP antibodies, RF). These labs are typically covered by insurance. I suggest you start here prior to undergoing highly specialized lab testing that may cost you hundreds of dollars.

AUTOIMMUNE SYNDROMES CAN LEAD TO CENTRALIZED PAIN

In a normal immune system, antibodies circulate and attack any foreign invader like an infection, toxin, or poison. Autoimmune diseases, on the other hand, occur in individuals whose bodies develop too many autoantibodies. *Autoantibodies* are antibodies that attack your own tissues. Your immune system, rather than protecting you from outside invaders, is now attacking itself. Depending on what syndrome you have, these autoantibodies will attack cartilage, nerves, glands, bone, blood cells, intestines, or organs. This leads to inflammation—and in those unfortunate enough to develop pain from their autoimmune disease—a form of centralized pain.

For those of you with autoimmune disease, you should seek treatment from a rheumatologist, in addition to doing the techniques in Part 2 of this book. You should also consider the Autoimmune Protocol Diet, which is not specifically described in this book. However, Dr. Terry Wahls[12] and Dr. Amy Myers have excellent books on using functional medicine to treat autoimmune disease. Both have witnessed incredible success stories and transformations in the patients who have followed their protocols. See Resources section.

Additionally, conventional medicine can be very effective in treating autoimmune conditions and may even be absolutely necessary in a flare. However, implementing the changes in Part 2 will allow you to heal your body, decrease flares, and possibly even wean off medications completely.

There are a number of autoimmune conditions that may be associated with chronic pain. Some of the more common ones are listed below.

Autoimmune Disease	Clinical Manifestations
Ankylosing spondylitis	Low back pain, sacroiliac joint arthritis
Ehlers-Danlos	Joint laxity, pain, or dislocation
Rheumatoid arthritis	Joint pain, loss of range of motion
Systemic lupus erythematosus	Generalized pain, joint pain
Psoriatic arthritis	Joint pain
Sjogren's syndrome	Muscle pain, joint pain

Note: If you have been diagnosed with fibromyalgia or chronic fatigue syndrome, I have seen some patients later be diagnosed with multiple sclerosis. Be sure to be evaluated by your primary care doctor or a neurologist if you have fibromyalgia to ensure you do not have early signs of multiple sclerosis, which can be diagnosed with imaging tests (MRIs).

SEVEN STEPS TO TREATING CENTRAL PAIN

Although there is likely a genetic predisposition to Central Pain Syndromes, I have found that the overwhelming majority of the time, symptoms can be controlled with lifestyle changes. Although genetics may have played a part in you being at risk for developing this syndrome, it is the factors your body has been exposed to thus far in your lifetime that triggered it. In other words, the reason you're in pain is largely due to environmental and lifestyle factors.

I have found the same seven factors contribute to the development and maintenance of Central Pain Syndrome. These factors lead to abnormalities in one's immune system and mitochondrial function, as well as cause brain inflammation, thus perpetuating the cycle of central pain. Due to this, your treatment plan must address and optimize all of these to achieve relief.

They are:

1. Dysbiosis (imbalance of gut microbes)

2. Nutritional deficiencies and food intolerances

3. Mental and emotional stress

4. Sleep

5. Hormonal imbalances

6. Exposure to and accumulation of toxic chemicals and/or toxic metals that alter the immune response

7. Inactivity due to severity of pain, which leads to more pain

DYSBIOSIS

It is estimated that around seventy percent of your immune system lives in your gut. Our gastrointestinal (GI) tracts house trillions of microorganisms, including bacteria, fungi, and viruses. This collective group integrates to form your microbiota. The gut microbiome plays a pivotal role in regulating your immune system. Issues arise when there is an imbalance in your gut bacteria—the bad bacteria outweigh the good bacteria. When you have a persistent imbalance of your gut's microbiota, you develop dysbiosis.

Chances are, your conventional medical doctor has done little to address your gut, when in fact, this is the key to so many underlying chronic diseases.

Small intestine bacterial overgrowth (SIBO) is when there is an excess of bacteria in the intestines. It is highly prevalent in those with irritable bowel syndrome and celiac disease. It can be diagnosed via lactulose breath testing (LBT).

This imbalance triggers changes in the junctions of our intestinal lining and leads to increased intestinal permeability or "leaky gut." Once your gut is "leaky," the bad bacteria from your GI tract can enter into your body, trigger an immune response, and cause issues elsewhere in your body. I see this condition often in those suffering from central pain, as well as in those who have taken anti-reflux medications for a long time.

Modern Western society has done a good job of destroying the healthy bacteria in our gut. Overuse of antibiotics and an increasing number of babies born via C-section have led to this. Babies acquire their microbiota from their mother during vaginal deliveries, so those delivered by C-section have delayed microbiota development. Researchers hypothesize this is the reason why we have so many more children with food allergies and asthma.[13]

In addition to this, we are living in an increasingly sterile world, where we are constantly using hand sanitizer and cleaning supplies to wipe away bacteria and other pathogens. I imagine that we may see an even further increase in these conditions as a result of the extreme cleanliness employed by the world during the COVID-19 pandemic.

Signs that you have dysbiosis include heartburn or gastroesophageal reflux disease (GERD), bloating, gas, digestive issues, constipation, and/or diarrhea. If you suffer from these symptoms or are taking chronic anti-reflux medications, I suggest you see a functional medicine practitioner. They can do lab tests to evaluate if you have SIBO and guide treatment with dietary changes, enzymes, and herbs to promote the health of good bacteria, evaluate if you need antibiotics or antifungal agents, and use probiotics and prebiotics specific to your needs. This is not a cheap route, as the stool culture analysis and supplements alone can cost hundreds of dollars.

For those who cannot afford to go this route, I suggest you start with reading and implementing the dietary changes in Chapter 9 and 10. You should still see a positive response, but it may take more time. If you find making these changes still has not cured your symptoms, then I suggest seeing a functional medicine practitioner.

YOUR MOUTH MICROBIOME

Your mouth is part of your GI tract and can also be a source of dysbiosis to the rest of your body. If you have periodontal or gum disease, you have inflammation in your mouth due to an overgrowth of bacteria. This bacteria triggers your immune system and can cause systemic diseases.

One sign of gum disease is your gums bleed when you brush your teeth or floss. Your gums may also appear red or be receding from the gum line. If untreated, this can lead to tooth loss. You should see your dentist regularly and adopt good oral hygiene by brushing and flossing twice a day. If necessary, your dentist can provide treatment for the dysbiosis via prescription mouthwashes or antibiotics. I also recommend using a Waterpik daily to clean your teeth. You can add an herbal antibacterial formula, such as Nature's Answer PerioBrite Cleanse, to the water in your Waterpik. It is important to remember that the mixture is not meant to be swallowed, and be sure to check the ingredients, as some may still enter into your bloodstream.

BUT I HAVE NO GI SYMPTOMS

It is possible you do not have any dysbiosis and have a perfectly healthy GI tract. Signs that you have no problems with your gut are: no stomach pain or discomfort after eating; having between one to three regular, solid, well-formed bowel movements a day; and never having bloating, cramps, or excessive gas. If you fall under this category, you do not need to worry about dysbiosis but should still consider making the dietary changes described below and in Part 2 to reduce your overall inflammation levels.

OPTIMIZE YOUR GI TRACT THROUGH YOUR DIET

Unfortunately, most of the time, patients with Central Pain Syndrome (CPS) have some level of dysbiosis in their gut. I recommend that all my patients with CPS implement dietary changes to optimize their microbiome balance and support their immune system.

A study by Galland demonstrated a tie between the gut and brain. They found dysbiosis, SIBO, and/or increased intestinal permeability (leaky gut) to be causes of brain and central nervous system inflammation.[14] The study reports ties between these conditions and fibromyalgia, chronic fatigue syndrome, and restless leg syndrome. It also postulated that our gut was responsible for our sleep and stress reactivity via a part of our nervous system known as the hypothalamic-pituitary-adrenal (HPA) axis. The HPA axis controls our body's hormonal response to stress.

People who consume diets high in fat, animal protein, and processed carbohydrates are more likely to have dysbiosis and leaky gut. This type of diet enables a balance of bad bacteria over good bacteria. Issues in your gut place you into a pro-inflammatory state. Since central nervous system inflammation is the driving force behind these central pain states, until you heal your gut, you will continue to suffer.

The quickest way to treat dysbiosis is to remove the harmful organisms. Conventional doctors, such as gastroenterologists, have typically done this by treating bacteria via antibiotics like rifaximin. Or if someone is found to have a fungal overgrowth, with an antifungal agent like nystatin.

Functional medicine practitioners tend to use herbs. Herbs have long shown to possess antimicrobial properties, and some herbs can effectively treat bacterial and fungal infections very well. A study by Chedid's group at Johns Hopkins found herbal treatment to be as effective as rifaximin (an antibiotic) for small intestinal bacterial overgrowth (SIBO).[15,16] The study used a proprietary blend of multiple herbs that is not commercially available, although there are some similar products on the market. I do not recommend taking herbs without the direction of a medical doctor because some can interact with other medications, cause liver or kidney toxicity, and affect pregnant women or their fetuses in harmful ways.

Although there are commercially available antimicrobial blends on the Internet, as well as at-home gut dysbiosis treatment programs from a variety of functional medicine doctors, I recommend you discuss these with your doctor rather than self-treat. The majority of the time patients do not have clinically significant leaky gut unless they have a true malabsorption syndrome, in which case you should visit with a gastroenterologist or functional medicine doctor for diagnosis and testing.

In most cases, doing an elimination diet followed by maintaining a gut-healthy diet will heal your GI tract and improve symptoms. See Chapter 9 and 10. Creating dietary changes to your GI tract is not a quick fix, and it can take ninety days to heal your gut. Be patient!

For those who do undergo treatment for dysbiosis, it is imperative to remember that if all that you do is take the antibiotics or herbs without removing the underlying triggers such as poor diet, stress, and toxins (i.e., alcohol and anti-reflux medications), your condition will recur as soon as you stop the medication.

In order to maintain a healthy gut, you need to consume an anti-pain, anti-inflammatory diet regularly. The general idea is to follow a modified Mediterranean-style diet: one that is rich in whole foods and contains minimal processed foods. By eliminating processed foods, you are eliminating dozens of harmful chemicals.

You need to eat a diet high in vegetables, fruits, nuts, seeds, and legumes (peas, beans, and peanuts) and very low in meat and saturated fats. Fill your diet with lean protein such as fish and poultry.

Avoid red meat and all processed meat. Studies have shown this type of diet restores the microbiota in patients.[17]

Remember also to add fiber to your diet. This means eating more fruits, vegetables, legumes, and whole grains and avoiding packaged goods. Maintaining this gut-healthy diet and drinking plenty of water is key to recovery.

NUTRITIONAL DEFICIENCIES

I typically do not recommend hundreds of supplements to a patient, and certainly you do not need to take all of these. However, due to the complexity of Central Pain Syndrome, many times more supplements are needed for it than for other conditions. Many of these only need to be taken for a period of time during the healing process and can be discontinued once you feel better.

A practitioner can help guide which ones can help your specific condition and also evaluate which ones may interact with your prescription medications.

Additional information, such as recommended doses and side effects, can be found in Chapter 11.

1. A high-quality multivitamin to make up for any gaps in your diet

2. Omega-3: EPA and DHA daily

3. Optional: Omega-6: 500 mg GLA from primrose or borage oil

4. Prebiotics

    Note: Prebiotics must be non-digestible by host enzymes, must be fermented in the GI tract by endogenous anaerobic colonic bacteria, and must be selective in stimulating intestinal metabolism. The use of prebiotics can lead to a shift toward good bacteria, decreased inflammation, and improved leaky gut.

Prebiotic supplements commercially available in the US are FOS, guar, lactulose, and inulin. However, instead of supplements, I generally recommend incorporating two prebiotic foods per day.

Warning: Ingesting prebiotics too quickly can lead to side effects such as stomach pain.

Prebiotic foods: Jerusalem artichokes, onions, leeks, garlic, bananas, soybeans, asparagus, eggplant, legumes (lentils, chickpeas), honey, or apples.

5. Probiotics to eliminate dysbiosis of the gut

Probiotics are live microorganisms that are ingested orally with the goal of restoring the balance of good to bad bacteria in your gut. Probiotics may contain a variety of microorganisms. The most common organisms found in probiotic formulations are bacteria that belong to groups called *lactobacillus* and *bifidobacterium*.

Ingesting probiotics may help with some symptoms of dysbiosis in the gut. However it is important to remember that probiotics have a very short-term effect of promoting healthy bacteria in your gut because ingesting them does not change your actual microbiome. Due to this, they must be ingested regularly and in a high-quality formulation. To truly repair your microbiome in the long-term, you cannot use probiotics as a magic bullet; you have to change your diet or get a stool transplant.

6. Coenzyme Q10

Patients suffering from mitochondrial dysfunction, particularly those with complex regional pain syndrome (CRPS), migraine headaches, restless leg syndrome, or fibromyalgia, are found to have defects in their mitochondria. As you recall, mitochondria are the powerhouses of our cells. They get rid of free radicals (toxins) and prevent cellular damage and inflammation. Often, patients with malfunctioning mitochondria are found to be deficient in coenzyme Q10 and may benefit from supplementation.

7. Riboflavin. Along with CoQ10, riboflavin can help support mitochondrial function.

8. Vitamin B_6 and Vitamin B_{12}. Supplementation may have a positive impact on mitochondria and also serve to protect neurons (nerve cells).

OPTIONAL SUPPLEMENTS

1. MTHFR mutation

Some individuals may suffer from a mutation in their MTHFR gene. This gene controls a process in our body called *methylation*. For those people who have clinically significant mutations in the MTHFR gene (not everyone with the mutation will have this), your body is unable to do some cellular processes properly, and the result is an elevated homocysteine level. This can lead to nerve pain issues, increased inflammation, and symptoms of fatigue. A homocysteine level can be tested easily by your doctor. If you are found to have a significant gene mutation, you may benefit greatly from supplementation with B_{12} and folate.

I recommend consulting with a physician rather than ordering these studies on your own because there are a lot of people with the abnormality that do not have clinical symptomatology. In that case, this would be an unnecessary supplement.

2. Alpha-lipoic acid

If you have signs of nerve pain (burning, tingling, numbness), particularly in the setting of diabetes, this can help.

3. Melatonin

Melatonin has actually been shown to affect pain perception.[18] A number of studies on Central Pain Syndromes, such as fibromyalgia, inflammatory bowel disorder, and migraines, demonstrate melatonin effectively reduces pain. These studies mostly used a 3 mg/day dose.[19]

SUPPLEMENT YOUR DIET NATURALLY

1. 5-HTP (tryptophan)

Tryptophan is an amino acid that can boost serotonin in the brain. Serotonin is a natural brain chemical that is vital in controlling pain, sleep, and mood. Lattanzio and his group investigated low serotonin levels in fibromyalgia patients.[20] His studies were based on the premise that fibromyalgia may be associated with low GI tract tryptophan absorption, which leads to low serotonin levels. One effective and natural way to boost serotonin levels is to increase tryptophan intake. Tryptophan as a supplement is no longer available in the United States due to cases of unusual blood disorders being linked to its use. 5-hydroxytryptophan (5-HTP) is still available, but 5-HTP is not a naturally occurring form of the amino acid. Due to this, I recommend the safest way to boost tryptophan is via diet (assuming these foods do not trigger your pain symptoms, which you will determine in Chapter 9).

a. Tryptophan can be boosted by eating the following foods: oatmeal, rice, or whole-grain bread in combination with poultry, fish, eggs, cheese, nuts, or tofu.

b. Certain foods and food additives affect the absorption of tryptophan and should be avoided. These are fructose, lactose, sorbitol, aspartame, and MSG.

c. Exercise boosts serotonin as well. You should aim to do at least twenty minutes of exercise daily.

2. Glutathione

    I recommend optimizing glutathione levels naturally because it is one of the most important antioxidants in the body. It can support immune function and reverse the effects of harmful toxins.

    You can increase your glutathione levels through diet. Excellent dietary sources of glutathione include spinach, avocados, asparagus, okra, broccoli, kale, and Brussel sprouts.

As you can see, food really is medicine!

FOOD INTOLERANCES

Common food sensitivities or food allergies that trigger central pain disorders are gluten, eggs, dairy, sugar, corn, and beef. Foods containing additives are also common culprits and include red wine, aged cheeses, processed meats (bacon, sausage), foods containing monosodium glutamate (MSG), tyramine, and nitrites.

I recommend you follow our elimination diet in Chapter 9, and be sure to eliminate the foods mentioned above, to identify your specific food sensitivities.

MENTAL AND EMOTIONAL STRESS

Meditation has been shown to decrease inflammation.[21] It has also been shown to be neuroregenerative with some studies demonstrating increased gray matter in those who practice meditation on a regular basis.[22]

I suggest implementing the mind-body techniques in Chapter 14.

Emotional traumatic experiences can often be tied to both Mind-Body Pain Syndrome and Central Pain Syndrome. In order to see if you have suffered any sort of emotionally traumatic experiences, please take the following questionnaire.

TRAUMATIC EMOTIONAL EXPERIENCES

1. Did a parent or adult you lived with often verbally abuse you (insult or swear at you)?

2. Did a parent or adult you lived with grab you, slap you, or physically abuse you in any way?

3. Did a parent or someone you lived with suffer from physical or verbal abuse?

4. Did you ever see your parents physically abused?

5. Were your parents divorced or separated?

6. Have you lost a parent or sibling?

7. Have you undergone a divorce or separation?

8. Did a parent or person older than you ever touch or fondle you in a sexual way?

9. Have you ever been raped?

10. Did you ever live with someone who suffered from a substance abuse disorder, like someone who abused drugs or alcohol?

If you answer yes to any of the questions above or feel you suffer from anxiety and/or depression, I recommend undergoing the program for Mind-Body Pain Syndrome (Chapters 5–6). Bear in mind, if you have experienced an emotional trauma, particularly in childhood, professional therapy is usually needed to heal from these life-altering events that can have lasting psychological and physical impact. Be kind and understanding to yourself.

SLEEP

Poor sleep is highly prevalent in central pain disorders. Please refer to Chapter 15 to optimize this. Optimal sleep is key to recovery.

HORMONAL

Hormone abnormalities are not only biomarkers for pain but avenues for treatment if one suffers from hormone imbalances.

In my experience, getting a patient's pain levels to zero is difficult to achieve if they have untreated hormone imbalances. The primary pain-controlling hormones are cortisol, dehydroepiandrosterone (DHEA), estrogen, pregnenolone, progesterone, testosterone, and thyroid-stimulating hormone. These hormones function to regulate the immune system, protect our cells, modulate our central nervous system, and even affect nerve function.[23],[24]

Of note, patients on chronic opioids are at particular risk for hormone suppression or abnormally low hormone levels. Patients on opioids should be checked for deficiency of the following hormones: testosterone, estrogen, pregnenolone, DHEA, adrenocorticotropin (ACTH), cortisol, and oxytocin.[25] Weaning off of opioids typically results in improvement of these hormone imbalances with time.

Research studying the impact of hormones on chronic pain elucidate one important fact: more women suffer from chronic pain than men. The noticeable gender disparity has led to further studies regarding the impact of hormones on pain. A clear mechanism has not been definitively described, explaining why women suffer disproportionately more chronic pain than men, but scientists hypothesize that it is primarily due to female sex hormones leading to an increased sensitivity to pain and different inherent immune systems in women versus men.

As we learned earlier in this chapter, the immune system impacts pain processing via the microglia, and studies demonstrate this pathway is impacted by sex hormones.[26,27] This leads to increased levels of both inflammatory and nerve pain in women as opposed to men. Sadly, despite biochemical research supporting a scientific reason for the elevated levels of pain in women as opposed to men, studies continue to show women's pain is undertreated in healthcare settings.[28]

Women's hormones predispose us to developing pain, but imbalances in hormones, such as those seen around menopause or menstruation, trigger periods of amplified pain.

To check for hormone imbalance, answer the following questions:

1. Do you feel your mood and energy swing from day to day?

2. Do you crave sugar or salt?

3. Do you have increasing levels of belly fat or are you obese?

4. Are you depressed or anxious?

5. Do you sleep poorly?

6. Do you have thin hair, dry skin, night sweats, or feel shaky?

7. Do you have issues with memory or concentration?

8. Are you sensitive to cold/heat?

9. Do you feel like your heart is racing?

10. Do you have issues with your sex drive?

Answering yes to any of these questions may point to a hormonal imbalance.

Without proper hormone balance, medications may not work as well, and pain remains difficult to treat. If this condition is suspected, a gynecologist or endocrinologist can check your hormone levels and provide guidance on replacement therapies. You should also investigate the dietary modifications, regular exercise, and stress reduction strategies described in Part 2 that can favorably change hormone levels. Be very careful who you are receiving hormone therapy from—there have been recent reports of various cancers resulting from pellet therapies and other forms of hormone replacement therapies. Check the credentials of the doctor you see. I personally recommend you try the lifestyle modifications first, as we are seeing more and more reports of cancers with long-term hormone replacement therapies.

Dr. Sara Gottfried and Dr. Anna Cabeca have books and online websites for treating hormonal issues from a holistic perspective (see Resources).

TOXINS

Toxins are often overlooked causes of central pain. Toxins can build up in your system, overload your mitochondria, and trigger a whole host of issues. You should assess your risk of toxic exposure to mercury, lead, and other biotoxins listed below.

Some questions to ask yourself to determine your risk of exposure are below. Make sure to think about your risk both at home and at your workplace:

1. I drink unfiltered water, well water, or water from plastic bottles.

2. I live in a building with poor ventilation or do not open my windows.

3. I live in an industrial area.

4. I live in a highly-populated area or big city.

5. I use chemicals often to clean.

6. I got my house exterminated.

7. I have silver (mercury amalgam) fillings in my teeth.

8. I eat large fish (tuna, shark, swordfish) more than once a week.

9. I am exposed to fumes often (gasoline, perfumes, new cars).

10. I dry clean my clothes often.

11. I use scented soaps/detergents or fabric sheets often.

Mercury has been linked to a variety of health issues, including chronic pain. Sources of mercury include dental work and fish. A functional medicine practitioner can do urine heavy metal testing if it seems you are at high risk for this. Dental fillings are often the source of mercury exposure. If you do have dental work with mercury, you should have those removed and consider seeing a functional medicine practitioner who can work to monitor your levels and give you additional herbs to help detoxify if necessary. You should avoid eating large quantities or regular amounts of mercury-containing fish.

In addition to mercury, other sources of toxins are pesticides, plastics, aluminum, cadmium, thallium, and arsenic.[29]

Another common biotoxin linked to this syndrome is indoor mold. Mold is different from mildew, although both are fungi. Mildew is a surface fungi you have probably seen in your bathrooms, kitchen, or basement. It is usually a patch of gray or white fungus on top of a moist area. It is easily treated with a cleaner and scrubbing brush. Mold, on the other hand, is usually black or green and is the result of a much larger amount of fungus. Mildew is usually easy to get rid of and causes at most some respiratory discomfort and/or coughing. Unlike mildew, indoor molds, particularly black molds, are responsible for neurotoxic illnesses that can manifest as brain fog, fatigue, poor sleep, digestive issues, and headaches. Risk factors for mold exposure include older homes, a known leak or flood, homes with basements that often have moisture, visible mold in basements (appears black and along areas where there is condensation, like furnace rooms), houses with flat roofs, and those in warm climates.

There are tests for mold. You can have your home tested by your city's health inspectors or mail a piece of your air filter to certain companies who test for mold. If you use a professional company to inspect your home for mold, be mindful that almost every home will have some level of mold in it, and that treating mold in your home is extremely expensive and not always necessary. Not everyone with mold in their home actually suffers from mold-induced illness. That is why if you can use a city health inspector, who does not have anything to gain financially, they can provide you with an honest recommendation on whether you need to invest in mold remediation. If possible, I suggest you take ten to fourteen days away from home, either at a relative's house or on a vacation, and see if the symptoms listed above resolve when away and return once you are home.

If you suspect mold-induced illness after taking time away from home, you should have yourself tested for mycotoxins to see if the mold is in fact causing you issues. After that, you should hire a mold remediation company to professionally remove the mold. It is important it is removed professionally because the agents used to kill mold are highly toxic and the area must be ventilated and secured per protocol to ensure everyone's safety.

Cholestyramine has been used as an off-label (i.e., not FDA approved) drug for treating mold disease, as has glutathione supplementation. I recommend removing the source, if possible.

Reference Chapter 16 for additional toxin removal strategies.

INCREASE YOUR OXYGEN

Hyperbaric oxygen therapy is a treatment where you inhale 100% oxygen in a hyperbaric (high pressure) chamber. The pressure is two to three times higher than normal air pressure. It is indicated for treatment of decompression illness, tissue-destroying infections, carbon monoxide poisoning, and gas emboli, to name a few. Although it has not been approved by the FDA for the treatment of complex regional pain syndrome (CRPS), fibromyalgia, or rheumatological diseases, it has been shown in small studies to be beneficial in these populations.[30,31,32]

I point this out not to say that everyone should run out and get an expensive treatment, but to emphasize that getting enough oxygen is important, and many of my patients are deficient in this simple area. I see it all the time. Many of my chronic pain patients take shallow breaths and rarely pause to take a deep breath and fill their lungs with air.

The solution doesn't have to be an expensive oxygen bar. It can be as simple as conscious, practiced breathing. I recommend you set an alarm every hour and do the 4–7–8 breath and breathing exercises described in Chapter 6. In between, try to be mindful of your breathing patterns. Try to recognize when you are shallow breathing and pause to take a deep belly breath as often as you can. For many of us, this alone will improve our symptoms.

HEAL WITH MOVEMENT

Regular aerobic exercises have consistently been shown to help decrease pain in Central Pain Syndromes. Studies show it decreases brain inflammation and promotes healing of our nervous system.[33] Numerous studies have demonstrated that exercise and physical activity improve CRPS and fibromyalgia, to name a few.[34]

It is possible that with Central Pain Syndrome, you suffer from some component of physical pain, such as "knots" (taut areas of muscle) or joint or spine issues. Please refer to Chapters 3 and 4 for diagnoses and specific exercises.

For the central pain patients with pain everywhere and an increased sensitivity to pain, I highly recommend tai chi, Feldenkrais, and somatic movement exercises. Please see the end of Chapter 6 for details.

HEALING FROM CENTRAL PAIN SYNDROME

Given how limited conventional medicine is thus far in finding medications that can effectively treat and reverse Central Pain Syndromes, I think the functional medicine approach described in this chapter is vital to improving quality of life. Please also use Part 2 of this book and follow the lifestyle guidelines recommended.

However, if you are curious about what Western medicine has that might be able to treat your symptoms, now or in the future, you can find potential treatments listed below.

CONVENTIONAL MEDICINE'S LIMITED OPTIONS TO EFFECTIVELY TREAT CPS

Prescription medications are commonly used for Central Pain Syndromes (CPS), but most are aimed at symptom management and not at reversing the underlying cause. Patients are traditionally given opioids, antidepressants, seizure medications, anti-inflammatories, and muscle relaxants in attempts to treat fibromyalgia symptoms, but often these provide little relief. Feel free to discuss these with your doctor, as they are routinely prescribed for many central pain conditions. I will review some alternative medical treatments for CPS below.

I present them here so you can discuss with your healthcare provider if they will benefit you or not.

GUAIFENESIN

Guaifenesin, otherwise known as Mucinex, is a cough syrup suppressant that some practitioners tout as the cure for fibromyalgia. Dr. Paul Amand has written about this treatment, and there are reports of one study showing its benefits. Please note that I was unable to find that report in the medical literature or any scientific evidence of its benefit in the treatment of fibromyalgia. As with many treatments, there are anecdotal reports of its success, but I cannot state that it is scientifically proven at this time.

KETAMINE INFUSIONS

Currently one of the more promising drug treatments to reverse Central Pain Syndromes, such as complex regional pain syndrome and fibromyalgia, is ketamine. Ketamine is a commonly used general anesthetic that has been around for many years. It works by blocking the glutamate receptor (NMDA), which is the primary receptor responsible for causing central pain. Overstimulation of NMDA receptors by glutamate leads to central sensitization, so you can imagine that blocking these should allow the nervous system to return to normal functioning. Ketamine has also been shown to help the brain repair neural damage, and intranasal ketamine has been shown to have a beneficial response in depression sufferers.[35] Ketamine is also a commonly abused street drug, known as Special K.

When used as a street drug, it can produce severe hallucinations and other untoward effects. When used in the clinical setting, it can help Central Pain Syndrome. It is important to note that ketamine is a highly dangerous drug and must only be administered under the supervision of a trained physician, as an overdose can lead to death.

There are a number of limitations to ketamine. As stated, it carries risks. These include, to name just a few, heart rhythm abnormalities and psychological side effects like nightmares and hallucinations. While at University of Chicago, I conducted a study with a former colleague of mine on ketamine infusions done in our outpatient pain clinic. Although we did find, on average, a fifty percent reduction in pain in our central pain patients, the pain relief was limited to three to four weeks.[36] Ketamine is not very effective orally and must be administered either intravenously or intranasally to get effective results.

Despite there being dozens of supportive studies, there remains a lack of high-quality randomized trials proving the efficacy of ketamine infusions, so the infusions have yet to gain insurance coverage, and remain very costly. One infusion can cost $500–$800. Like I stated earlier, this is an anesthetic drug, used to put people to sleep under general anesthesia for surgeries. Only doctors skilled at airway management should be administering ketamine in an office setting (i.e., anesthesiologists, intensive care unit doctors, or emergency medicine physicians).

We also do not know the long-lasting effect of using ketamine. Studies have shown repetitive use of ketamine causes negative impact on memory and cognition.[37]

POSSIBLE FUTURE TREATMENTS

We have yet to identify medications that can completely reverse the microglial activation that leads to Central Pain Syndromes. You may recall the microglia being the immune system cells of our nervous system. The most promising treatments so far are naltrexone and minocycline, which can down-regulate microglia and decrease nervous system inflammation.[38,39]

LOW-DOSE NALTREXONE

Naltrexone is a medication that blocks the effects of opioid medications such as morphine, heroin, and codeine. It works by competing with these drugs at the same receptors in the brain. It blocks the effects of opioids.

Several studies suggest naltrexone can benefit those with Central Pain Syndrome such as fibromyalgia, complex regional pain syndrome, multiple sclerosis, and Crohn's disease.[40]

Unfortunately, as of now, it is only for off-label use and is not FDA approved for these conditions. You can only get it by prescription from a compounding pharmacy. It is usually $30–$70 per month out of pocket. It is typically well tolerated, has a good safety profile, and has no abuse potential.

MINOCYCLINE

Minocycline is actually a tetracycline antibiotic. It has been shown to have anti-inflammatory and microglial-modulating activity. However, adequate studies for its use in central pain are yet to be done.

PRACTITIONERS YOU COULD BENEFIT FROM

Although conventional medicine is very limited in affordable, effective options for Central Pain Syndrome, knowing which practitioners to partner with and what changes you can make will help you on your path to healing.

1. Your primary care doctor and a functional medicine doctor are key to your recovery.

2. A rheumatologist is necessary if you suspect autoimmune issues.

3. Cognitive therapists: Talk therapy is important, but you need to find a therapist specialized in biofeedback/CBT. See Resources.

4. Interventional pain physician: They can help provide relief via procedures if the pain is unbearable. Some of these include ketamine infusions, lidocaine infusions, spinal cord

stimulators for complex regional pain syndrome (CRPS), and various injections. If you have a diagnosis of CRPS, I strongly recommend seeing a pain physician as soon as possible because sympathetic nerve blocks done early in the course of the disease have more success at breaking the pain cycle and reversing the central pain process. In my own clinical experience as well as a number of case studies, ketamine infusions done early on have more success in breaking the cycle.

Central Pain Syndrome is extremely challenging to treat, but I have seen many patients successfully treat CPS using the techniques described in this chapter. Even if you cannot eliminate your pain, reducing it to manageable levels through various treatment approaches can greatly impact your quality of life.

PART 2

REPAIR AND RESTORE

CHAPTER 8

INTEGRATIVE HEALING OF MIND—BODY—SPIRIT

"The doctor of the future will give no medicine but will interest his patients in the care of the human body, in diet, and the cause and prevention of disease."
—Thomas Edison

George was a seventy-one-year-old firefighter who was released from duty on medical leave after pain developed following a fire where a woman he attempted to rescue died. When I evaluated him, I realized this trauma had led to symptoms of post-traumatic stress disorder (PTSD), but that he also had poor lifestyle habits, as well as muscle imbalances that had led to sacroiliac joint pain and a lot of stress-induced tension in his neck and shoulders leading to chronic headaches. I knew his case did not fit simply into one syndrome and that we would have to approach his case step-by-step. Up until this point, not one of the seven physicians he saw had suggested cognitive therapy to address the PTSD as a trigger for pain. When we combined cognitive therapy, lifestyle changes, physical therapy, and injections to address his physical pain, he drastically improved. He had been living with increasing pain for twenty years, and after only six months, we were able to wean off his muscle relaxants and other pain medications that left him in a fog all day.

THE WAY IN WHICH WE LIVE

At one time, our ancestors were hunters and gatherers, spending their days scouring for food. When they would encounter a predator or prey, their nervous systems would spring into fight-or-flight mode, and once hunting was done, their systems would relax once more. We now live in a different world, one in which we have successfully eliminated most external threats to our daily lives. Why is it, then, that we are suffering the most?

A 2006 national survey of patients undergoing treatment for chronic pain reported over half of patients felt they have little or no control over their pain.[1] That is an extremely large number of people finding no answers with our current healthcare system.

Unfortunately, our pioneering developments, advanced technologies, and increasing farming capabilities have opened the door to modern-day threats that have led to endless amounts of chronic pain and chronic disease. We live in a sedentary world that has exposed us to man-made toxins and food that is chemically enhanced and nutritionally deficient. This relatively "easy" life has led us to be unable to handle stress the way our ancestors did, so we now remain in a constant fight-or-flight mode. We have created the perfect recipe for a chronic pain storm.

Certainly, some portion of risk for developing pain is due to genetic factors. However, we are now learning the impact of epigenetics on chronic pain development. Epigenetics refers to the science behind how your environment and behaviors can change the way your genes are expressed. In other words, genetic factors work in tandem with environmental influences to affect the expression of chronic pain.

For example, studies have shown women to be genetically more prone to developing chronic pain, but that this is heavily influenced by environmental factors, lifestyle habits, and lifetime experiences to produce epigenetic changes affecting one's pain perception.[2,3] The exact molecular mechanisms driving epigenetic changes are still being studied, but scientists propose environmental toxins, diet, medications, and emotional stressors alter cellular processes like DNA methylation, RNA changes, and cellular protein expression that are leading to the development of chronic pain.[4,5]

Understanding these factors helps us understand why one person may have a disc bulge and recover within a few weeks, while another person might be plagued with unrelenting pain for years. The reason for this is simple: One was predisposed (through genetics, lifestyle, or other external circumstances) to developing the cycle of pain, while the other was not.

Part 2 aims to teach you how to live well and decrease the environmental and lifestyle factors that could elevate your chronic pain risk.

It was shocking to me when I discovered the incidence of chronic pain is greater than that of heart disease, diabetes, and cancer combined. Chronic pain is a preventable chronic disease. And it can be effectively treated utilizing a comprehensive, individualized treatment algorithm, as outlined in this book.

Let's review what leads to the development of the chronic pain cycle. There are two phases.

PHASE 1:

Low Levels of Systemic Inflammation + Toxic Burden + Muscle Imbalances from a Sedentary Lifestyle + Constant Stress → Risk of Developing Chronic Pain

PHASE 2:

Elevated Risk Due to Phase 1 + Triggering Factor (Emotional Trauma Causing Severe Mental Stress or Physical Injury or Surgery) → Chronic Pain Cycle

To expand on the example of two patients with bulging discs—although they both experienced the same triggering factor (an injury), their bodies were in different states going into this injury. Each one had a different foundation makeup as a result of their lifestyle choices from Phase 1. One of the patients was a highly active individual who regularly did yoga, practiced meditation, and generally followed a Mediterranean diet. The other was a type A, high-stress individual who barely had time to eat breakfast or lunch and rarely exercised. As you can already imagine, each one's response to the injured disc was very different. I have seen it countless times in my practice. Patient one is far more likely to heal and be back to themselves within twelve months, whereas the second patient would have a far more complicated and less successful course.

The reason my program is not a quick fix is that the end product of Phase 1 took years to develop. Years of poor exercise, diet, and exposures to toxins and low-level inflammation is not going to be reversed overnight. It is going to take months of your new lifestyle to entirely reverse Phase 1, but it is possible. The body can do remarkable things when given the right tools and fuel.

I hope that when you see it this way, you can understand why chronic pain is a systemic disease and why simply correcting the symptoms (i.e., shaving off the disc bulge with a minimally invasive back surgery) is not going to permanently heal your pain.

Unless you address *all* the factors above, it is going to be near impossible to achieve a long-term, pain-free life.

Part 2 of this book is going to teach you the second half of my ninety-day program to repair and reverse those years of damage we began repairing in Phase 1. By doing this, we can have long-lasting improvements with the therapies you are concurrently doing from Part 1 of this book. It won't be easy, but I hope you will try to implement as many positive lifestyle changes as you can afford to. This portion of the program should be a minimum of forty-five days because that is the time it will take to begin to see improvement. However, to continue to see results, you need to implement the lifestyle changes long term.

What is included in the Part 2 forty-five-day plan? It consists of five basic components:

1. A nutritional/diet plan including a twenty-one-day elimination diet to identify sensitivities and triggers, followed by a long-term anti-pain, anti-inflammatory diet for the remainder of the program

2. Supplements you can take based on your specific condition to complement the changes made in your diet

3. Lifestyle changes, including a daily exercise regimen, mindfulness practice, and optimal sleep routine

4. Identification and removal of environmental toxins in your life

5. A pain treatment toolbox with tips, products, and techniques that you can use to self-manage your pain

You do not need to follow each of these steps in sequential order. Some people will want to start with the easiest steps first and build confidence. Others may want to tackle the harder things first. Many will need to plan the elimination diet out carefully, so it will come later as they read the other chapters and implement what works for them. The goal is to do your best and realize that *any* improvement in these areas will have profound benefits. Perfection is not the goal, and it may even be a stumbling block toward progress.

LEARNING TO CHANGE

Any lifestyle habit change requires consistency and dedication. Doctors often tell their patients to eat better, sleep better, and exercise, but patients are often given no actionable steps to get there and don't know where to start. Use this book as your roadmap.

If at any time you begin to feel overwhelmed with the effort, cost, or time required, please refer to my Quick Guide in the "Final Thoughts" chapter at the end of this book.

Let's dive in and tackle these plans of action one by one!

CHAPTER 9

ELIMINATE THE
INFLAMMATORY SOURCE

When my second daughter was born, she had horrific reflux and colic. However, her colicky symptoms were not just limited to the evenings. She cried for hours on end, day after day. This, of course, impacted her sleep. She would sleep for forty-five minutes at best and then would wake up screaming inconsolably again. And since she was exclusively breastfed, I did not sleep either.

In an attempt to help her, I researched various natural remedies and implemented them, to no avail. By the time she was six weeks old, I knew her condition needed medical attention. We visited her doctor, and she confirmed my suspicion—my daughter had a food allergy causing gastrointestinal reflux. Aware that I tried to avoid all medications if possible, the doctor told me that if I wanted to continue to nurse her, the best thing for her was an elimination diet for me. So I began a strict elimination diet.

By the end of week three, my daughter drastically improved, and I continued the diet. At the end of month two, the most incredible thing happened. For the first time in almost four years, I could walk barefoot around my house. The swelling in my foot that had been plaguing me for years, causing me to limp every day at work, was gone. My food "sensitivity" ended up being dairy, something that had never bothered me before. Eating dairy had given me zero symptoms outside of this foot swelling.

Before I knew it, I was able to return to Zumba class. Up until the diet, I had managed to obtain seventy percent relief through stress reduction and correcting physical imbalances, but thirty percent of my pain persisted until I implemented the elimination diet. The elimination diet finally broke my pain cycle. To this day, my foot pain has never returned.

An elimination diet is the foundation of true healing. While other methods may be easier, like costly food sensitivity tests, a three-week elimination diet is mandatory to detox and reset your gut and body, as well as identify food triggers specific to you.

It is particularly beneficial for those with heartburn, irritable bowel syndrome, seasonal allergies, acne/eczema, bloating, fatigue, hives, migraine headaches, autoimmune conditions like rheumatoid arthritis, and fibromyalgia. So let's get started.

WHAT IS AN ELIMINATION DIET?

An elimination diet is a twenty-one-day restrictive diet that involves removing all potentially problematic foods, allowing your body to heal and symptoms to subside. After this period, you then slowly reintroduce foods into your diet one at a time to see which foods trigger your symptoms.

Very important: This type of diet is *not* meant to be a permanent diet.

WHY SHOULD I DO THIS?

Some people have true allergies, meaning they eat a food and quickly develop a rash or vomiting or even have trouble breathing. However, many of us have hidden food sensitivities—that is what the elimination diet aims to uncover. Like allergies, food sensitivities are a type of immune reaction, but a much slower one. Sometimes these symptoms do not develop until several hours or even a few days after you have eaten the food, which makes it very hard to identify the culprit. Food intolerances can produce a multitude of symptoms, the most important one being continuous levels of inflammation. This can present as bloating, gas, sleep issues, congestion (sneezing or coughing), decreased energy, muscle aches, joint pain, depression, anxiety, and acne. The best way to identify these intolerances and how your body is reacting to different foods is to do an elimination diet. And best of all, it's free!

WHO SHOULD NOT DO THIS?

The elimination diet described in this chapter is not for those experiencing any of the following:

1. Allergies or severe digestive symptoms. These severe symptoms include:

   a. Multiple loose bowel movements a day.

   b. Undigested food in your stool.

2. A GI condition, such as inflammatory bowel disease, SIBO (small intestinal bacterial overgrowth), or irritable bowel syndrome. For these individuals, I recommend doing an elimination diet under the direction of a functional medicine or GI doctor, because you will need to repair your gut first, which will involve the addition of botanicals, digestive enzymes, and medical foods. If you do fall into this category and cannot afford a functional medicine provider, discuss the diet with your primary care doctor.

3. An eating disorder.

4. Daily alcohol consumption. If you are a daily alcohol drinker, consult with your physician. Depending on how much and how frequently you drink, you may have severe withdrawal symptoms if you suddenly stop drinking.

5. A daily prescription medication routine. Also anyone on *any* prescription medications—particularly those on blood thinners, diabetes medications, psychiatric medications, or

heart medications or those with liver issues or kidney disorders—should not introduce any dietary changes without first discussing them with your doctor. The detox diet can cause changes in your blood sugar as well as changes in how medications are metabolized, so it is very important to discuss with your doctor first.

HOW TO DO THE ELIMINATION DIET

The diet has two phases.

Phase 1: The detox phase is to calm the immune system and heal your gut. During this phase, you eliminate all triggering foods. Some elimination diets recommend you juice, drink green smoothies, and/or drink pureed vegetable soups alone to give your gastrointestinal (GI) system a break from having to digest solid foods. You can do this method if you like. However, I don't usually recommend a full liquid diet because juice diets can be shocking to some systems and also very challenging to maintain. Because of this, I recommend simply eliminating all the triggering foods.

Phase 2: During the reintroduction phase, you will begin a structured food challenge to see which foods you react to.

ELIMINATION DIET: PHASE 1

For the first twenty-one days, you will eliminate the following foods. In order to successfully do this, you will need to read the labels of everything you eat. For most people, this means preparing the majority of their food at home rather than eating out at restaurants or at friends'/family's houses. This is why I recommend you plan the elimination diet for a period of time where you have no travel plans, holidays, or important celebrations.

AVOID:

- Gluten-containing grains (barley, rye, wheat)

- Dairy

- Soy, soy products, and peanuts

- Corn

- Eggs

- Sugar such as corn syrup, cane sugar, fructose, glucose, sucrose, and dextrose

- Alcohol, coffee, tea, soft drinks

- Peanuts

- Pork, beef, processed meats, shellfish

- Food additives (MSG, artificial food coloring, guar gum, artificial sweeteners)

- GMOs (which are *genetically modified organisms* commonly added to our foods. Look for non-GMO on your labels)

- Preservatives (such as BHA, BHT, nitrites, sulfites, to name a few)

- Dyes (will typically have a color listed such as Red 40, Yellow 5)

- If you have arthritis or joint pain of any kind, eliminate nightshade vegetables (tomatoes, potatoes, eggplants, peppers, cayenne, chili peppers)

YOU MAY EAT: Dairy alternatives (unless they contain soy or peanut products), fish, fruits, game meats, gluten-free whole grains (amaranth, buckwheat, quinoa, or rice), healthy cold-pressed oils, legumes (except soy, peanuts), nuts (not peanuts), poultry, seeds, an abundance of veggies

Some people have even better results if they eliminate all meat and fish for the second and third week. This is optional.

The table below can be used as a reference.

	Allowed Foods	Foods to Avoid
Fats	Cold-pressed oils like olive oil, flaxseed, walnut, hazelnut, pumpkin seed, sesame, or sunflower oil	Butter, shortening, peanut oil, margarine, mayonnaise, any processed or hydrogenated oil
Beverages	Filtered water, decaffeinated tea, pure fruit juice or mineral water, coconut water	Soda, soft drinks (even Diet), alcohol, coffee, tea, caffeine, sweetened juices
Sweeteners	Brown rice syrup (gluten-free), pure maple syrup, agave nectar, stevia, xylitol, monk fruit extract, coconut sugar/extract	White/brown sugar, high-fructose corn syrup, honey, corn syrup
Spices & Condiments	Vinegars (check grain source), wasabi, mustard, horseradish, all spices	Chocolate, ketchup, soy sauce, BBQ sauce, relish, condiments
Fruits	Strawberries, citrus, pineapples, apples, apricots, avocados, bananas, blueberries, cherries, grapes, kiwis, mangos, melons, nectarines, pears, peaches, plums, raspberries	Grapefruit, sweetened fruits (canned/frozen), and sweetened fruit juice

Vegetables	All fresh, raw, steamed, grilled, sautéed, roasted, or juiced vegetables that aren't on Avoid list	Creamed vegetables, tomatoes and tomato sauce, corn
Starch	Rice (white, brown, wild), potatoes, oats (gluten-free), quinoa, tapioca, millet, buckwheat, amaranth	Corn, gluten-containing products, wheat, barley, rye, kamut, spelt
Legumes	All legumes, lentils, and peas	Soybeans, tofu, tempeh, soy milk, soy sauce, or anything with soy protein
Nuts & Seeds	All nuts except peanuts	Peanuts, peanut butter, and peanut oil
Meat & Fish	All fresh or frozen fish (except shellfish)—wild better than farm raised, chicken, turkey (organic and hormone-free is best)	Tuna, swordfish, shellfish, beef, pork, cold cuts, hot dogs, sausage, canned meats
Dairy Products	Milk substitutes like rice milk, oat milk, nut milk	Milk, cheese, cottage cheese, cream, butter, ice cream, yogurt, non-dairy creamers, soy milk, and eggs

DIETARY PAIN TRIGGERS

Many of us are sensitive to gluten, even if we do not test positive for celiac disease. Gluten has been the culprit for a lot of pain conditions, including joint pain, back pain, arthritis, and other ailments.[1] Some reports have found up to forty percent of people without celiac disease are sensitive to gluten and can present with headaches, fatigue, and nerve, bone, muscle, or joint pain. When eliminating gluten, look for hidden sources like your lotions, medications, supplements, and shampoos.

Dairy is a big pro-inflammatory food and can lead to a variety of pain complaints.[2] Despite what commercials have told us, you do not need cow's milk. Lactase is converted into glucose, a sugar, which triggers inflammation. Additionally, milk products can contain contaminants that range from hormones to pesticides. You can protect against osteoporosis by getting your calcium from dark leafy green vegetables and strength training.

Sugar is another big culprit. Sugar is not only highly addictive, but also leads to insulin resistance, heart disease, obesity, and inflammation. Be sure to read labels carefully, as sugar can come in many hidden forms, such as corn syrup, high-fructose corn syrup, dextran, dextrose, diastase, fructose, fruit juice concentrate, galactose, glucose, agave nectar, maltodextrin, maltose, mannitol, maple syrup, sorbitol, sucrose, and treacle.

DIETARY TRIGGERS FOR SPECIFIC CONDITIONS

GAS/IBS/GI SYMPTOMS

If you predominantly suffer from irritable bowel symptoms, chronic diarrhea, lots of bloating or gas, you may be sensitive to FODMAPS. FODMAPS include beans, soy products, apples, pears, peaches, plums, nectarines, broccoli, cauliflower, cabbage, onions, garlic, and green onions. If you fit into this category, I recommend cutting out all FODMAPS and adding them back one by one.

MIGRAINE HEADACHES

A study by Grant[3] showed when headache sufferers eliminated certain triggering foods, over eighty percent became headache-free. These migraine triggers were wheat, orange, eggs, tea, coffee, chocolate, milk, beef, corn, cane sugar, and yeast. If you suffer from migraines, you should eliminate all of these and then add them back one by one to see if they trigger your symptoms.

ARTHRITIS/AUTOIMMUNE CONDITIONS

Those with arthritis and autoimmune conditions are likely to find benefit by eliminating nightshade vegetables. These include eggplants, tomatoes, potatoes (not sweet), bell peppers, and spices from peppers like cayenne and paprika.

Many other chronic pain conditions have been tied to food sensitivities, including arthritis, chronic back pain, interstitial cystitis, muscle pain, joint pain, temporomandibular disorders, and fibromyalgia.

This diet will help identify your individual food triggers.

HELPFUL TIPS

- Soup is an excellent way to get lots of herbs, spices, and vegetables. Batch cook a huge amount and freeze it in a mason jar for times you are hungry or do not have time to prepare a meal.

- Smoothies are a great way to load up on green leafy vegetables. Consider adding some hemp or chia seeds. Smoothies are an excellent way to get your daily fruits and vegetables and fight cravings.

- Make sure you are getting enough nutrients. This is why doing an elimination diet under a physician's guidance is best, as they can supplement your diet with medical foods.

- Make sure to take a good quality multivitamin with vitamin B_{12}, magnesium, and vitamin D_3, as well as probiotics and a fish oil supplement. See Chapter 11 for additional details.

- If you are not doing this with medical foods, you can make a daily smoothie with 1-2 scoops of pea protein powder. Be sure to read the labels to ensure the protein powder does not have any ingredients from the "Foods to Avoid" list.

- Before you start, wean off caffeine for three weeks. You do not want to be simultaneously weaning off caffeine as you are going through the detox process.

- In the week leading up to the diet, start eating a clean diet. Avoid alcohol, caffeine, processed foods, and refined sugars while focusing on quality proteins, good fats, and lots of greens. This will make the detox a little less shocking to your system.

- Exercise has many beneficial effects, including increasing oxygen delivery to tissue and improving bowel function. However, during the elimination diet, you may need to cut down on strenuous activity. If you exercise and feel fatigued, take a break. I do not recommend starting a new exercise program during these three weeks.

- Screen your medications, toothpastes, and personal care products for any ingredients on the "Foods to Avoid" list.

- Write the "Allowed Foods" on a notecard and keep it with you at all times. That way you always have a good reference for what you can and cannot eat. If you downloaded the Companion Guide (see front of book), there is a chart you can print in there.

REMEMBER: EAT AS MUCH AS YOU WANT!

One plus of the elimination diet is there is no caloric restriction—you can eat as much of this nutritious food as you want! The goal is not weight loss, but to support and restore a healthy microbiome, use phytonutrients to heal the gut, reduce toxic burden, identify food triggers, and reduce inflammation.

Remember, the goal of this diet is not to lose weight. When you follow our dietary recommendations in the next chapter, you are more likely to lose weight. The elimination diet is a short-term challenge, similar to Whole 30. It is a very restrictive diet, and it is not recommended you continue it for over three to four weeks.

SIDE EFFECTS

I will warn you, most people do not feel great during the first few weeks of the elimination diet. The detox phase is challenging. To minimize these side effects, I recommend you first wean off of caffeine and begin eating healthy in the three weeks leading up to the elimination diet. This will make the diet go much more smoothly for you.

Side effects you may experience as your body detoxes are the following: runny nose, brain fog, headaches, fatigue, flu-like symptoms, muscle aches, skin rash, sweating, and GI distress such as gas, bloating, and changes in stool consistency.

Buffered Vitamin C (1 gram, 1–2 times a day), fiber supplements, and peppermint tea can help abate GI distress. If you are feeling lightheaded, it may be due to hypoglycemia (low blood sugar), so make sure to eat enough protein and frequent meals.

PHASE 2: REINTRODUCTION

After the first twenty-one days, you should be feeling better. Your fatigue, joint pain, and headaches should have improved. If they have, then you can continue with the reintroduction. If they have not, continue the elimination diet for one more week and be very prudent with checking to see if things you are eating actually do have some hidden sources from the "Foods to Avoid" list.

If you are still experiencing symptoms after all of this, you should visit with a functional medicine practitioner or nutritionist who can give you further direction. You may need to get tested for small bowel intestinal overgrowth (SIBO) and receive specific treatment to enable the elimination diet to be more effective.

It is very important in this phase that you keep a symptom journal. This is part of the Companion Guide you can download (see Free Gift offer at the start of the book).

In this journal you will keep track of the food reintroduced and note if it caused any of the following symptoms during the three days you reintroduced it.

Did the Food Cause...	Yes/No
GI distress	
Headaches	
Muscle pain	
Decreased energy	
Joint pain	
Rash	
Other	

It is crucial you introduce no more than one food item at a time in the order below and that you allow three days before introducing another food item. Each newly introduced food should be eaten during at least two of your three daily meals for three consecutive days. If you begin to react before the three days are finished, stop eating that particular food. Wait until the reaction subsides, which typically takes one to two days, and then move on to the next food.

To try to keep this simple, I am only including the main culprits for pain. Please refer to the conditions above to see if you should be reintroducing additional foods one by one.

Day 1–3: Dairy

Day 4–6: Wheat/gluten

Day 7–10: Corn

Day 11–13: Eggs

Day 14–16: Tomatoes. If you eliminated nightshades, add them back after these three days.

Day 17–19: Shellfish

Day 20–22: Coffee

Day 23–25: Soy

Day 26–29: Peanuts

If you have not reacted at all to anything up until this point, you may be sensitive to the following less common dietary pain triggers and may want to continue the three-day reintroduction of the following: alcohol (especially red wine), caffeine, MSG, aspartame, onions, corn, citrus fruits, nitrites, meat, chocolate, and apples.

MOVING FORWARD

For many, completely eliminating a food they are sensitive to is very challenging. I recommend the 80/20 rule when it comes to food sensitivities. Eighty percent of the time, do not eat that food. Some people will react so negatively that they will need to avoid it one hundred percent of the time. However, for others, the 80/20 rule should be sufficient to keep your pain at a minimum and eliminates some of the stress that could come (and be counterproductive) with being hypervigilant about every bite you put in your mouth.

CHAPTER 10

FOOD AS THE
FOUNDATION OF WELLNESS

"The food you eat can either be the safest and most powerful form of medicine or the slowest form of poison."
—*Anne Wigmore*

June was a fifty-two-year-old female who visited me after a referral from a friend. I was her last resort and fourth pain doctor. She had horrific pain in her left thigh and ankle. She limped in with a walker. She was also plagued with migraines, bloating, gas, and lack of energy. Her medical file took me over an hour to dig through. There were dozens of injections, imaging studies, and notes from visits to various specialists, including surgeons, rheumatologists, neurologists, and podiatrists. She had spent over $10,000 on various treatments, from stem cell injections to acupuncture treatments—none of which gave her any relief. She felt hopeless and depressed that she would have to live her entire life like this.

I gave her instructions for an elimination diet followed by maintenance with a plant-based, whole-food diet. Within two months, her migraines and energy issues had resolved. By three months, her foot and leg pain had vanished—and she ditched her walker. She was able to regain strength through physical therapy and adopted a mindfulness program. She maintains the diet until today with continued success and resolution of symptoms.

BEST ANTI-PAIN DIET

The reality is that there are dozens of diets out there—and many that seem contradictory can help the same pain condition. For example, I have seen fibromyalgia patients benefit from being Paleo and others benefit from going one hundred percent vegan.

Diet is a very personal choice. There are cultural or economic reasons why one might choose one diet over another. If I wanted to go through each and every diet and the supporting evidence, I would fill three textbooks. Not only that, but if I truly were to dig through all the literature out there, for every article I found promoting one diet, I would find another one saying that diet was completely wrong. So instead I am going to discuss healthy dietary habits that work for most, if not all, chronic pain conditions and chronic diseases.

No matter what diet you choose, I highly recommend you check out the Cronometer app. It is an excellent nutrition tracker app for your smartphone that enables you to track your diet and uncover if you are potentially deficient in up to eighty-two micronutrients. This could save you hundreds of dollars on expensive diagnostic nutritional lab testing.

WESTERN DIET EFFECTS

Generally speaking, the average Western diet contains way too many refined carbohydrates, not enough essential fatty acids, and low levels of fiber. The standard American diet has been shown again and again to lead to states of inflammation.[1] In fact, scientists have coined a term, *inflammaging*, which refers to how our bodies are showing increasing levels of inflammation as we age. Inflammaging is a chronic condition that results from having elevated levels of pro-inflammatory compounds. These compounds are interleukin-6 (IL-6), tumor necrosis factor-alpha (TNF-alpha), and interleukin-1 beta (IL-1β) system.[2]

Obesity has long been shown to lead to low levels of inflammatory markers. It is known that these fat cells release chemicals promoting inflammation and lead to inflammatory conditions such as heart disease, diabetes, and chronic pain.[3]

When inflammatory chemicals remain elevated through diet and/or obesity, we alter our gut microbiome, which leads to chronic inflammation. Chronic inflammation leads to many chronic pain conditions. There is also an increased incidence of diseases such as type 2 diabetes, cardiovascular disease, neurodegenerative diseases like Parkinson's, and cancer.[4]

It has repeatedly been shown in animal studies that the standard American diet, high in processed foods, refined sugars, omega-6 polyunsaturated fatty acids, and carbohydrates, triggers elevated inflammation and poorer healing from injuries when compared to an anti-inflammatory diet.[5]

It has also been shown that a healthy diet, particularly when coupled with exercise, can actually change the composition and diversity of your gut microbiome.[6] In fact, healing your gut is the best way to enhance your systemic immune function and combat chronic pain, since the majority of pain issues are tied to underlying rates of chronic inflammation.

WHAT TO EAT

An ideal diet should consist of plenty of fruits and vegetables, whole grains, nuts and seeds, legumes, minimal to no dairy products, and fish. Not all of us can be vegan or vegetarian, nor do I recommend that for everyone.

Although you do not need to follow a formulaic diet, I have found that it's helpful for some patients to have a plan. If you do like specific diets, there are three I recommend for chronic pain. I like (1) Dr.

Andrew Weil's anti-inflammatory diet, (2) the whole food plant-based diet (Dr. Neal Barnard is an excellent resource), or (3) the Mediterranean diet with minimal to no red meat intake.

You can check out the resources section for recommended books on diet.

ANTI-PAIN DIETARY RECOMMENDATIONS

Remember that these are recommendations for a healthier, pain-free you. Also remember that every step is a good step. You will probably not be able to incorporate each of these suggestions into your diet tomorrow. There may even be some that you cannot implement until resources or income permit. However, don't let that stop you from taking some steps now! Each thing you do will help your body reduce inflammation and decrease your pain. The purpose of this list is not to overwhelm, but to fully inform. Do what you can and add to it as you are mentally and financially able.

1. General diet: Emphasize fruits, vegetables, nuts, seeds, berries, healthy fats, and lean sources of protein.

2. Limit intake of caffeine, alcohol, processed foods, dairy, sugar, and red meat. If you do eat beef, limit to one to two times per month and only grass-fed. Ideally, you eliminate all of these as much as possible.

3. Eliminate soda. Replace with sparkling water or flavored water.

4. If you found any food sensitivities in Chapter 9, eliminate those foods.

5. Eat the rainbow every day! Eat five to nine servings of fruit and five to nine servings of vegetables daily. Using the table below, be sure to eat produce from each of these categories every day. The phytochemicals and antioxidants in these various vegetables can help fight cancer, boost your immune system, and reduce inflammation.

Eat the Rainbow!

Red	Tomatoes, watermelons, guavas
Orange	Carrots, yams, sweet potatoes, mangos, pumpkins
Yellow	Oranges, lemons, papayas, peaches, grapefruit
Dark Green	Spinach, kale, collards
Light Green	Broccoli, brussels sprouts, cabbage, onions, asparagus
Blue	Blueberries, grapes, plums
Purple	Grapes, berries, plums
Brown	Whole grains, legumes

6. Consume healthy fats. No trans fats. Emphasize omega-3 fats.

7. Eat a low-glycemic, low-sugar diet.

8. Use spices liberally. Some anti-inflammatory spices include basil, black pepper, garlic, ginger, cloves, cinnamon, and turmeric.

9. Drink green tea!

10. Use the 80/20 rule. Eat well eighty percent of the time; and give yourself a break twenty percent of the time.

11. Intermittent fast. This can alter your gut microbiome and have great health benefits like improved cognitive function, weight loss, decreased inflammation, and improved mitochondrial function.[7] Try to fast twelve to fourteen hours every other day (most do 8:00 p.m. to 10:00 a.m.). During this

time, you can only consume black coffee, plain tea, and water. Fasting is not for everyone, so listen to your body. For women, in particular, fasting may affect your thyroid hormones and cause you to miss a period. For those who experience these issues or have autoimmune thyroid disorders, consider a milder fast, like two to three times a week for ten to twelve hours. If you feel worse with fasting, it may not be for you.

12. Eat one to two prebiotic foods every day (asparagus, cabbage, chicory, garlic, Jerusalem artichokes, and leeks, to name a few)

13. Consider supplementing your diet with the following: a high-quality multivitamin, alpha-lipoic acid, omega-3 fatty acids, and probiotics to synergistically work to reduce stress, pain, and inflammation. See Chapter 11.

14. Eliminate processed foods to avoid the formation of dietary advanced glycation end-products (AGEs), which are known to lead to a number of chronic diseases, as well as decrease your overall omega-6 levels, which are pro-inflammatory.

15. Try to drink eight to ten glasses of water a day. Drink clean water. www.EWG.org has a Tap Water Database to search for water pollutants by zip code, as well as recommendations on what are the best water filters based on your area's contaminants.

16. Eat plenty of fiber.

17. Eat fresh, local produce that is in season—more vegetables than fruit. If eating fruit, try to stay away from the ones with higher levels of sugar, like grapes and bananas, and choose low-glycemic fruits such as cherries, grapefruit, and berries.

18. Increase glutamine, a non-essential fatty acid naturally found in foods such as cabbage, lentils, beans, tofu, spinach, and fish.

19. Eat meals with others. Community is key. Try to make it a device-free meal.

20. Sweets are reserved for special times, not every day.

21. Start reading labels. Try to only eat items with under five to six ingredients. Fewer is better!

22. Detox from added sugar. If you are really struggling, eat some fruit or a small amount of 80–100 percent dark chocolate.

TIPS ON EATING ORGANIC ON A BUDGET

When you can, try to eat organic fruits and vegetables. Here are some cost-saving tips:

1. Buy local produce, or seasonal produce, and freeze for later. Buy organic produce when on sale and freeze what you don't use. You can check online for what produce freezes best. You can freeze greens and fruits within three days of purchasing to use later in smoothies.

2. Purchase grocery store brands.

3. Look for grocery store coupons in the mail, online, or on the store's app.

4. Grow an herb garden.

5. Check out www.EWG.org for the Dirty Dozen and Clean Fifteen lists to see what to splurge on in terms of organic foods versus what to skip.

6. Purchase just what you need from the bulk section in grocery stores—nuts, spices, etc.

7. Make homemade granola and snacks.

8. Make homemade baby food in bulk. I did this and loved the savings!

9. Look for organic coupons online at www.allnaturalsavings.com or www.organicdeals.com.

10. Buy frozen. Frozen fruits and vegetables tend to be cheaper, especially if something is out of season.

11. Grow your greens inside. You can use empty plastic produce containers (punnets) from your old groceries to grow them. This website tells you how to do this indoors for cheap. Greens, sprouts, and herbs can all be grown indoors without a garden: https://veganorganic.net/windowsill-gardening/. You can buy non-GMO seeds from www.sowtrueseed.com.

12. Buy and keep bananas separated from one another—they spoil slower.

13. Keep all organic citrus fruits in the fridge—they will last up to one to two weeks longer.

14. Do not wash organic dark leafy greens or berries until they are ready to consume.

15. Store herbs, spring onions, and asparagus upright in a large glass filled with an inch of water. You can freeze many herbs too!

As we conclude this chapter, I want to bring an important point to your attention. Please remember to be kind to yourself as you make a change to your diet. Orthorexia is an increasing problem as we are inundated with loads of nutrition information everywhere we look. Orthorexia is a term for a negative condition that results due to obsessive thoughts and behaviors around pressure to maintain a perfect, healthy diet. It may lead to a real psychological disorder, and the effects can be detrimental.

Many chronic pain patients already suffer from anxiety and depression and may be vulnerable to developing anxiety surrounding all the changes they want to make. Remember to do your best, but that you do not need to live your life to the extreme. Aim for good, clean eating seventy to eighty percent of the time. That means one to two days a week, give yourself a break.

CHAPTER 11

FIGHTING PAIN THE NATURAL WAY: SUPPLEMENTS THAT WORK

Thirty-year-old Sally came to my clinic with multiple areas of neuropathy (nerve pain). She had a long-standing history of carpal tunnel syndrome that had failed injections and bracing. More recently, she had developed numbness and tingling in her leg after a Pilates class three weeks prior. From the history, I figured out this happened after she used a Pilates ring that had compressed a nerve on the inside part of her lower thigh, known as the saphenous nerve. She had been doing Pilates for years and never had issues, so she couldn't even fathom how an uneventful Pilates class could have led to nerve damage. She had spoken to some friends about it and even her primary doctor, who had all convinced her she had sciatica, or a pinched nerve in her spine. So why would an otherwise healthy thirty-year-old get persistent numbness from a five-minute exercise?

Many medications commonly taken can cause vitamin deficiency leading to neuropathy, or nerve pain. In Sally's case, it was the Prilosec she took for acid reflux. Be sure to always review possible side effects of your medications. Fortunately, with Sally, it was easy to diagnose. I didn't even wait for her labs and recommended she start a B_{12} supplement until we weaned her off Prilosec through diet and lifestyle changes. I also added alpha-lipoic acid supplements to aid in recovery. Two weeks later, all of her symptoms were gone, including the numbness in her hands (her carpal tunnel symptoms). She discontinued the supplements but continued with our lifestyle modifications, which kept her reflux at bay.

Supplements are by no means a replacement for a healthy diet. No supplement will fix poor diet and lifestyle habits. However, even with a perfect diet, due to the poor quality of our food supply and high load of environmental toxins, most of us will need a daily supply of some supplements to fill the gaps. Studies have shown deficiencies in individuals eating a standard American diet, and health benefits with supplementation.[1] For most people, a high quality, bioavailable multivitamin (MVI), vitamin D_3, methylation factors (folate, B_6, and B_{12}), and omega-3 fatty acids (EPA and DHA) will be all that you need. You may be able to find a multivitamin that contains a lot of these. If you have GI symptoms, you may also benefit from a probiotic.

Please remember supplements should not be started without first discussing them with your doctor. The doses in this chapter are provided as a guide based on the doses used in the studies referenced. Specific supplement dosages should be determined by your doctor, as there are a number of prescription medications that interact with supplements.

This chapter will show, based on your condition, what additional supplements may benefit you. If you follow the diet recommendations in Chapter 10 at least eighty to ninety percent of the time, you will not need to spend hundreds of dollars on supplements. I also do not typically keep patients on supplements forever. Some are used during the detoxification and healing phase, and then only a handful of supplements are continued long term. Always be sure to discuss supplements with your healthcare provider, as you may not need to continue all of them.

To provide an additional cost-savings option, I have included dietary sources of the supplements below. I always recommend getting your vitamins through diet rather than supplements.

The goal of this book is a cost-effective approach to self-management of pain, so this is not an exhaustive list of every possible supplement.

Note: Any and all vitamins, herbs, and botanical supplements must be discussed with your doctor, as some can interact with your other medications. The following dosing guidelines do not apply to pregnant and nursing mothers or children. Those individuals should not take any supplements without discussing with their doctors, as many can be harmful. The doses listed are daily max doses, so be sure to check all your vitamins so you do not take too much.

CHOOSE SUPPLEMENTS WISELY

Our supplement industry in the US is not regulated by the FDA, so not all supplements are the same quality.

1. Look for manufacturers who use GMP (good manufacturing practices).

2. Look for third-party analysis for verification of active ingredients and contaminants.

   a. Brands displaying labels by Consumer Lab, NSF International, or US Pharmacopeia are great because these nonprofit groups have verified contamination-free products and GMP.

3. Visit this website: https://ods.od.nih.gov/Health_Information/ODS_Frequently _Asked_Questions.aspx, as well as those listed in the appendix to research your supplement brands.

4. Only use supplements that have scientific basis to them and a long history of safety.

MULTIVITAMIN (MVI)

Look for a multivitamin that provides 75%–150% daily value for vitamin A, B_1, B_2, B_6, B_{12}, C, D, E, K, folic acid, and niacin as well as selenium, copper, magnesium, iodine, and zinc. It is best to take your multivitamin with a meal to enhance absorption.

TURMERIC (CURCUMIN)

How it works: Anti-inflammatory (inhibition of PGE2, leukotrienes, and nitric oxide)

Uses: May help depression, osteoarthritis, pain after you have surgery, inflammation, and autoimmune conditions like rheumatoid arthritis.[2,3]

Dietary sources: Turmeric is a spice commonly used in Asian food that is derived from the root of the turmeric plant.

Doses: 1–2 grams daily dried root, or 500–1,000 milligrams daily in capsules

Caution: Avoid in cases of gallbladder issues; can cause GI distress (heartburn, nausea). Avoid if taking blood thinners, diabetic medications, or tacrolimus.

VITAMIN B₂ (RIBOFLAVIN)

How it works: Vitamin B_2 plays a critical role in important metabolic processes in the body, such as normal cell function and energy production by the powerhouses of our cells (mitochondria).

Uses: It can be used in Central Pain Syndromes, particularly migraine headaches.[4]

Dietary sources: milk, eggs, meat, nuts, and green vegetables.

Doses: 200–400 milligrams daily

Caution: Usually pretty safe but can cause diarrhea in some. Avoid if taking tetracycline antibiotics.

FOLATE

How it works: Folate functions as a coenzyme for many important reactions in our body. It helps in making DNA and controlling important genetic material in our bodies. It is also responsible for a very important chemical reaction: the conversion of homocysteine to methionine. If this reaction does not take place, you can get elevated homocysteine levels, which can trigger heart disease and neurological issues such as nerve pain.

You may have heard of a methylenetetrahydrofolate reductase (MTHFR) gene mutation before. The MTHFR enzyme is critical for metabolizing folate and keeping your levels of homocysteine in check. If you have the mutation, you may have high levels of homocysteine and low levels of other vitamins due to problems with your body's chemical reactions. This can cause issues such as anxiety, depression, chronic pain, and fatigue. It can also affect your body's response to certain medications. Those who have MTHFR mutations and take drugs that affect folate metabolism, such as methotrexate, may be more likely to experience toxicity. The presence of the mutation can be tested on www.23andme.com. It is important to note that not all people with the deficiency have clinical symptoms as a result of the deficiency. If you do decide to undergo testing, discuss with your doctor first.

Uses: Those with clinically significant MTHFR deficiency, inflammatory bowel disease, anxiety, nerve pain, or depression may benefit from folate supplements.[5,6]

Dietary sources: Spinach, liver, asparagus, and brussels sprouts have the highest folate level, but nuts, beans, and eggs are also good sources.

Doses: Doses can be 400–800 micrograms daily.

Caution: Can interact with methotrexate, seizure medications, and sulfasalazine. Avoid if you have anemia. (Discuss with your doctor.)

Tip: Metanx ® is a prescription vitamin with L-methylfolate calcium (an active form of folate), B_6, and B_{12} that brings relief to many patients with neuropathy, or nerve pain.

VITAMIN B6

How it works: Plays a role in pathways that decrease nerve pain signals (via synthesis of serotonin and GABA, which are chemicals known as neurotransmitters).

Uses: May help with nerve pain, elevated homocysteine levels, menstrual cramps, carpal tunnel syndrome, depression, and brain function.[7,8]

Dietary sources: Bananas, garbanzo beans, chicken, fish, oatmeal, potatoes, spinach, and avocados.

Doses: 50–100 milligrams per day. Takes up to three months to see results.

Caution: Can interact with blood pressure, heart medications, or seizure medications. Can cause nausea, vomiting, abdominal pain, and headaches.

VITAMIN B12

How it works: Vitamin B_{12} plays a role in key processes, including nerve and nervous system function, proper red blood cell formation (the cells that transport oxygen), and DNA synthesis.

Uses: Nerve pain or elevated blood levels of homocysteine.[9] It is important to note that a lot of medications cause B_{12} deficiency, and I have seen marked improvement in nerve pain, which typically presents as burning, shooting pain, simply by supplementing with vitamin B_{12}. Some common medications that can cause B_{12} deficiency are metformin, proton pump inhibitors for acid reflux, and colchicine. Regular alcohol use can lead to B_{12} deficiency as well.

Dietary sources: Most dietary forms of B_{12} come from animal products, including fish, meat, poultry, eggs, milk, milk products, or fortified cereals. Most vegans and vegetarians not eating fortified foods should supplement.

Doses: 1,000 micrograms, with at least half coming in the form of methylcobalamin

Caution: Can increase risk of blood vessel narrowing if you have had a stent placed. Be careful if you have megaloblastic anemia or Leber's disease. Can interact with a number of medications. At recommended doses, it is usually well tolerated.[10]

GINGER

How it works: A natural anti-inflammatory. It works by affecting the inflammatory cascade, through inhibition of cyclooxygenase and lipoxygenase enzymes. Inhibiting these enzymes inhibits the synthesis of leukotrienes (inflammatory chemicals that cause pain).

Uses: Joint pain, menstrual cramps, muscle pain, arthritis.[11,12,13]

Dietary sources: Dried ginger may be a better anti-inflammatory than fresh ginger.

Doses: 500–1,000 milligrams per day

Caution: Can cause GI distress. May interact with blood pressure and blood thinner medications.

OMEGA-3 (FISH OIL)

How it works: Anti-inflammatory. Acts by competitively inhibiting the enzymes cyclooxygenase and lipoxygenase.[14,15,16]

Uses: Joint pain, inflammatory pain, nerve pain.

Dietary sources: Fish. Note: Be careful about contamination of fish as well as contaminants in the supplement. Unfortunately, fish oils are often highly contaminated with waterborne pollutants, and it is challenging to find a good product. Due to this, young children and pregnant women should avoid taking large amounts of fish oil or eating lots of fish. When buying fish oil supplements, look for bottles that say they come from small fish. Small fish are less likely to be contaminated with toxins than larger fish because the larger fish eat smaller fish and the toxin levels add up. Find a high-quality brand with the guidelines recommended at the start of the chapter, and look for a seal that states its manufacturer has either removed or tested for contaminants.

Doses: At least 2 grams daily of the fish-derived omega-3 fatty acids EPA and DHA. For severe chronic pain, you may need higher doses.

Caution: Can cause heartburn or fish burps. High doses may cause gastrointestinal (GI) distress. Can cause bleeding in those on blood thinners. May interact with blood thinners, blood pressure medications, and birth control.

PROBIOTICS

How it works: Probiotic supplements can have varying amounts and types of bacteria in them. The best combination of bacterial strains to formulate the ideal probiotic has not yet been delineated. The one that has been studied the most is *Lactobacillus casei*. Your best bet is either to eat probiotic foods regularly or to take a probiotic with mixed organisms per capsule for the ninety days you are undergoing this program. Most do not need to be on probiotics indefinitely.

You should look for one that gives you ten to twenty billion mixed organisms per capsule. Most will have different strains of lactobacillus and bifidobacterium species. These are the most studied. Look for one with at least four to five different strains. They can be taken either once or twice a day per the serving instructions on the bottle.

They can be in capsule form or powders. Be sure to check the label to see if the formulation needs to be refrigerated or not.

Uses: Can help with digestion, anxiety, depression, and arthritis.[17,18,19]

Dietary sources: Fermented foods are great sources of probiotics. For example, yogurt, kefir, sauerkraut, tempeh, kimchi, kombucha.

Doses: Ten to twenty billion organisms taken on an empty stomach or with food twice a day.

Caution: Can cause gas, diarrhea, bloating.

MAGNESIUM

How it works: Works by mediating brain and nervous system inflammation, and also works as a smooth muscle relaxant.

Uses: May help with headaches, muscle pain, anxiety, insomnia, fibromyalgia, chronic fatigue, restless leg syndrome, and diabetic nerve pain.[20,21,22]

Dietary sources: Magnesium can be found in beans, tree nuts, brown rice, seaweed, and green vegetables.

Doses: 300–600 milligrams daily. Many wonder what form of magnesium to take. According to the NIH website, small studies demonstrate magnesium in aspartate, chloride, lactate, and citrate forms is absorbed more completely and is more bioavailable than magnesium oxide and magnesium sulfate.

Caution: Can cause diarrhea. Be careful, as lots of important medications for heartburn and rheumatoid arthritis, antibiotics, warfarin (blood thinner), and blood pressure medications are just some of the medications that can interact with magnesium.

Tip: For migraine sufferers, the combination supplement MigreLief has been beneficial.

ALPHA-LIPOIC ACID

How it works: Alpha-lipoic acid is an antioxidant produced naturally in the body and obtained via dietary sources.

Uses: Can help with nerve pain, particularly in diabetics, and painful bladder syndrome and can reduce body weight.[23,24] Can possibly help with (though there is less evidence to support its use for) carpal tunnel syndrome, neck/back pains, and migraines.[25]

Dietary sources: It is found in yeast, yams, carrots, red meat, spinach, broccoli, organ meats, and potatoes.

Doses: 300–600 milligrams daily

Caution: Use with caution if on blood thinners or thyroid medications. In diabetics, it may lower blood sugar.

VITAMIN D

How it works: It has many roles and is very important! Vitamin D plays a role in cell growth, neuromuscular and immune system function, and reduction of inflammation.

Uses: Can help with osteoarthritis, muscle pain, headaches, diabetic nerve pain, and obesity.[26,27,28]

Dietary sources: Vitamin D is found in sockeye salmon, fortified milk, fortified orange juice, egg yolks. Most people obtain some vitamin D through exposure to sunlight , but for most it is not enough. In supplements and fortified foods, vitamin D is available in two forms, D_2 (ergocalciferol) and D_3 (cholecalciferol). They differ chemically only in their side-chain structure, but work in similar ways. There is not a definitive consensus on which one is superior, but Vitamin D_3 appears to be more potent.

Doses: Dosage should depend on your lab results, so work with your doctor. It is usually 1,000–2,000 IU (international units) daily unless you have very low levels. Your doctor should guide you on dosing.

Caution: Vitamin D toxicity can cause weight loss, heart arrhythmias, and damage to the heart, blood vessels, and kidneys. May increase calcium levels in patients with a number of conditions and may interact with numerous medications, including cholesterol and heart medications.

Note: Vitamin D enhances absorption of calcium, so it's usually best to take these supplements together.

MELATONIN

How it works: Many people are familiar with the effect of melatonin for sleep, since melatonin is a hormone naturally produced by our bodies that regulates the sleep-wake cycle. However, melatonin also regenerates axons (critical parts of a nerve cell) and reduces oxidative stress (toxin buildup).

Uses: It has been shown to improve sleep and improve symptoms in a variety of chronic pain and inflammatory syndromes, including jet lag, work-shift sleep disorders, fibromyalgia, headache, IBS, low back pain, migraine, and rheumatoid arthritis.[29,30] For those taking beta-blockers (blood pressure medications), check with your doctor because many beta-blockers can significantly decrease melatonin levels. These patients may experience difficulty sleeping due to this and would improve with supplementation.

Doses: 0.5-5 milligrams sixty minutes before bedtime

Caution: Ideally melatonin is used for under four to eight weeks, although studies have demonstrated benefit up to twenty-four weeks.[31] It can interact with a number of medications, including blood thinners and those for diabetes, blood pressure, and seizures. It may cause headache, dizziness, or nausea.

COENZYME Q10

How it works: Coenzyme Q10 is a fat-soluble compound with a chemical structure similar to vitamin K. It plays a key role in muscle cell energy production. CoQ10 improves energy, augments the immune system, and acts as an antioxidant.[32]

Uses: It improves headaches by enlarging blood vessels via the chemical compound nitric oxide. It can also be used to reduce muscle pain and for migraine headaches, diabetic nerve pain, and centralized pain syndromes such as fibromyalgia.[33] Statins, commonly-used cholesterol-lowering medications, have been shown to reduce the amount of naturally occurring CoQ10 in the body. For patients taking statins, supplementation might reduce the risk of muscle pain.

Dietary sources: Primary dietary sources of CoQ10 include oily fish (such as salmon and tuna), organ meats (such as liver), and whole grains. Most individuals obtain sufficient amounts through a balanced diet, but supplementation may be useful for the above conditions.

Doses: 50–300 milligrams daily

Caution: Can cause GI distress at higher doses. May interact with blood pressure and blood thinner medications.

N-ACETYL CYSTEINE

How it works: It plays a role in decreasing pain signals by serving as a potent antioxidant and increasing glutathione levels in the body. Glutathione plays a vital role in detoxification and other important pathways that keep you healthy.

Uses: May work for nerve pain, mood disorders, centralized pain syndrome, and neurodegenerative diseases.[34] Shows anti-inflammatory properties.[35]

Dietary sources: Cauliflower, broccoli, and asparagus. Vegetables with a high sulfur content, such as green leafy vegetables, also lead to higher glutathione.

Doses: 300–600 milligrams daily

Caution: Can cause GI side effects. May interact with blood thinners, blood pressure, and antimalarial medications.

ACETYL L-CARNITINE

How it works: Carnitine plays a critical role in energy production. It transports fatty acids to the mitochondria, our energy factories, so they can be converted into fuel our bodies can use. It is also involved in removing toxins from the mitochondria and is found in our muscle tissue. In most people, the body makes sufficient carnitine. But for some, it can be a much-needed supplement.

Uses: Nerve pain, depression, muscle pain, fibromyalgia.[36,37]

Dietary sources: Is found in meat, fish, and dairy products primarily and in lesser amounts in asparagus or whole wheat bread.

Doses: 1,500–2,000 milligrams daily

Caution: Can cause GI side effects. May interact with blood thinners, particularly coumadin.

GLUCOSAMINE AND CHONDROITIN SULFATE

Many people use glucosamine and chondroitin for osteoarthritis (OA), particularly of the knee. Smaller studies and some good-quality studies have shown some benefit[38] for improving knee arthritis pain. However, larger trials and other analyses found no effect.[39] Additionally, there is debate as to whether glucosamine sulfate versus glucosamine hydrochloride is more effective.

Due to these inconsistencies in the literature, I did not include information on this supplement. I recommend you do your own research and discuss with your healthcare provider, as some trials have shown it can help knee arthritis.

CONCLUSION

It is very tempting to consider purchasing every single supplement that you hear could possibly help your condition. However, I urge you to remember that if you follow the diet and lifestyle recommendations in this book, you likely will not require loads of supplements to heal your pain. Use this chapter as a guide to begin a conversation with your doctor on what supplements may be helpful complements to your diet.

CHAPTER 12

POSITION YOURSELF FOR SUCCESS

WRITTEN WITH REBECCA PAULIN-LISTON, PT, RYT

At the start of the COVID-19 pandemic, I shut my clinic down for about two months, along with many other healthcare facilities. My practice shifted to telemedicine, or online consults, for the first time ever. A long-standing patient of mine, a twenty-six-year-old teacher, called me with severe neck and shoulder pain. She was desperate for an injection, but given the lockdown, I was not performing any.

We had a virtual visit where I was able to make a diagnosis that her pain was due to neck and shoulder muscle spasms related to her positioning during the day and other ergonomics due to her working from home. I was able to walk her through what pillow to use, how to station her desk, what stretches to do, and what topical treatments to use, and she was able to completely resolve her pain without procedures or prescription medications.

This was the case for several patients with similar pain complaints during the pandemic.

How we sit, eat, sleep, and stand throughout the day plays a huge role in whether our bodies are in pain or pain-free. This chapter will focus on optimizing ergonomics and posture so we can treat current pain issues and prevent them from occurring.

1. **Pillows/Mattresses**

   - Choose pillows and mattresses carefully. See Sleep Chapter 15.

2. **Avoid Texting Neck**

   - When holding your phone, hold it out in front of you and not down in your lap. Try to keep your neck in a neutral position. If you are holding your phone up, try to keep your elbows at the side of your body, and switch hands throughout the day.

3. **Chairs/Desk**

   - Keep your mouse close to the side of your computer. Remember to keep elbows close to you so your arms are bent and close to your side. This prevents adding tension to your shoulder muscles.

   - Try to use standing desks or limit time sitting. Do not sit for longer than twenty minutes.

4. **Wrist Position**

   - If you spend a lot of your day typing, or wear a tight watch, have wrist or hand burning pain or numbness, you need to do the carpal tunnel stretch more frequently. For those watch wearers, loosen your watch and alternate wrists.

   - Keep your wrist neutral while typing.

5. **Texting Thumb**

   - I see an increasing number of thumb arthritis and tendonitis issues of the hand directly related to smartphone and iPad/tablet usage. Try to utilize apps where you can text by voice. Also alternate hands or fingers.

6. **Seat Cushions/Lumbar Support Cushions**

- Sit with a pillow placed in the curve of your lumbar spine (low back). This is right above your belt line. You can use a regular pillow, but remember to adjust it for each chair. It is important that it is comfortable and allows you to be in the correct position where your posture is straight and not slumped, but your low back is supported and comfortable.

7. **Driving**

- When driving, at stoplights, place your hands behind your head and hold it in this gentle stretch for thirty seconds.

- You can also do your chin tucks during a stoplight. See appendix.

- Use a lumbar support cushion and consider a seat cushion if you have buttock or pain down your legs.

- Drive with your hands at 4 p.m. and 8 p.m. instead of 10 p.m. and 2 p.m. as we are taught. It puts less strain on your shoulder muscles.

8. **Supportive Braces/Belts**

- Outside of SI Joint belts as mentioned in Chapter 4, I do not usually recommend back braces unless you are pregnant (and should use specific braces designed for your stage of pregnancy) or unless you just had surgery or a spine fracture. If you have muscle imbalances and wear a brace, you will worsen them due to disuse.

9. **Footwear**

- Supportive footwear is key.

- Make sure shoes are not too wide or too narrow.

- Sorry, ladies, high heels are terrible for your feet. If you must wear heels, try wedges that provide more support. Wearing heels too long can cause calf tightness and plantar fasciitis, among other issues.

- Try varying your footwear day to day.

- Try to have someone look at you when you are barefoot on a hard surface. Check if there is any space under your arch. If you have a flat foot, you need arch support.

  o If your arch is flat but you are able to "make an arch" by raising the inner edge of your foot off the ground with your big toe on the ground, you have a flexible flat foot. For this, you can try Powerstep insoles off Amazon ($27) or custom orthotics through a reputable podiatrist or physical therapist using your insurance. I recommend trying the cheaper ones first because even if you use your insurance, custom orthotics can cost hundreds of dollars.

  o If your arch remains flat no matter how much you try to raise it or support it, you most likely have a fixed flat foot, and your foot needs more gentle support— try something "accommodative" like Vasyli full length green insoles (Amazon $55).

10. **Lifting Heavy Objects**

- Stand with a wide base of support and the object between your feet if possible (if the object is awkward to handle see below).

- Bend at your hips and knees keeping your back straight— pretend you are sitting your hips back into a chair—and lower your chest and arms to reach the object.

- Bring the object to you while straightening your legs, pressing into your feet to activate your hips.

- Exhale as you lift to help engage your core.

11. **Carrying Items**

- Alternate which arm is doing the carrying throughout the day.

- For women, I have seen lots of shoulder issues arise out of heavy bags worn over one shoulder. Try rolling suitcases, a backpack, or carrying your handbag at your side alternating arms.

12. **Canes/Assistive Walking Devices**

- For those of you who use a cane, adjust the top of the cane to rest right at the level of your wrist crease when you are standing straight with your arm six inches away from your side and forward.

- Try to choose a cane, such as the Campbell Cane, that allows you to stand upright.

- Trekking poles. Some people prefer these adjustable walking sticks that can be height adjusted and often have an ice tip for use in winter. They are also meant to be used in both arms, which is helpful to maintain the normal rhythm of your gait.

- If you use a walker, use it as little as possible and keep correcting your posture every fifteen minutes by standing straight and deep breathing with neck up, shoulders back. Make sure the top of the walker where your hands rest is adjusted to the level of your wrist crease when you are standing straight and tall with your arms slightly out to your sides.

CHAPTER 13

WHOLE BODY STRENGTH
AND WELLNESS

WRITTEN WITH REBECCA PAULIN-LISTON, PT, RYT

Jake, a thirty-two-year-old real estate agent, came to see me in the clinic with back pain. He already had an MRI, which read as normal outside of some mild degeneration. When I spoke to him, I realized he lived a very stressful lifestyle and did absolutely no physical activity. By the time I saw him, he had been treated by the conventional medical system and given a week of oral steroids. He had been taking ibuprofen every six hours for four months. Nothing had worked. He was still in pain.

Fixing his pain was easy because it was physical pain resulting from years of inactivity and various weaknesses. He said he did not have time for physical therapy. I put him on an exercise program similar to the one in this chapter, and his pain disappeared in two months. We were fortunate he was referred to see me by a friend, as his primary doctor had not referred him to anyone but a surgeon. We were also fortunate that his MRI was normal and that he had not undergone an unnecessary surgery for an unrelated finding on his MRI.

As we learned in Chapters 3 and 4, the majority of chronic pain in the world is actually a result of muscular imbalances. In order to live well, we need to constantly work to return our body to a state of balance.

BENEFITS OF EXERCISE ON PAIN

We have come to accept that underlying low levels of inflammation and inflammatory chemicals lead to a lot of our chronic diseases. Regular physical exercise has long been shown to be anti-inflammatory in nature. Epidemiological studies have shown that physical inactivity is associated with systemic low-grade inflammation and that physical activity and fitness are associated with a reduction in inflammatory biomarkers known as *cytokines*.[1]

DAILY EXERCISE REGIMEN

1. Do strength training twice a week. Our exercise regimen below counts, but feel free to modify it for your level or condition. As you grow stronger, incorporate exercises that use resistance bands or light weights to further strengthen the muscle groups.

2. For cardio, I recommend a whole-body exercise for thirty minutes, one to two times a week, that promotes coordination, such as swimming or aerobics. Find something you enjoy.

3. You should also aim to incorporate HIIT (high-intensity interval training) for fifteen to twenty minutes twice a week. HIIT training can greatly help with losing weight and improving cognition, and it supports mitochondrial function in addition to many other health benefits.

4. If you are too deconditioned to do HIIT training, then replace it with walking at least 8,000–10,000 steps a day.

5. Try to go outdoors every day. Outdoor activities like cycling or hiking are great for both physical and mental benefits. Walking has many benefits, including decreasing pain, strengthening your bones, and improving your mood. I highly recommend involving your whole family in some technology-free time outside.

EXERCISES TO DO SO YOU DON'T END UP IN MY CLINIC

Note: For those who were diagnosed with specific imbalances in Chapter 4, the exercises in that section are important to work on daily or every other day as instructed. The following exercises are designed as a total body approach to prevent further/future problems from developing, and these would be good to add in a couple times per week in addition to your other regimen.

For those who do not have any physical imbalances, follow this program.

Any exercises not described below are in the exercise appendix.

TIPS FOR SUCCESS

1. Be mindful of your posture throughout the day. Think of Figures 2 and 3 from Chapter 4.

2. If you are spending your day at a desk, it is important to do this stretch once an hour or whenever your shoulder blade area or neck feels tight.

    Take your hands and place them on the top of your head. This puts those overstretched muscles into an unstretched position and allows them to reset. Hold this position for sixty seconds and take this as an opportunity to work on your deep breathing.

3. Stretches can be done daily, but be sure not to overstretch.

4. Strengthening exercises should be done every two to three days.

5. Working on balance and whole-body stability is key. It is important to continue to work on balance as we age. Try to improve stability by balancing on one foot every day (or several days per week). This allows you to strengthen, but also to keep track of how balanced your muscles are. You can

balance on one foot on a thick rug (or bath mat) and/or close your eyes to make this more challenging. Some of my patients find doing this while brushing their teeth kills two birds with one stone. You can also use a wooden wobble board for 3-5 minutes a day, such as the Yes4All Board on Amazon.

6. It is important to work on keeping your bones strong and healthy while you age. To do this, make sure you walk daily or do some form of weight-bearing exercise.

ANTI-PAIN EXERCISE PROGRAM

See appendix for any exercises not described here.

1. Deep breathing. Lying on your back with your knees bent, take a deep breath in with your hand on your belly. You are trying to lift your hand up with your breath in. On your exhale, allow your belly to flatten, drawing your navel toward your spine. You may feel like your stomach muscles are "hugging in" or that you are engaging the muscles from one pelvic bone across to the other. This is the deepest layer of your core muscles that helps you stabilize your spine and your pelvis. Repeat this ten times with your breath.

2. *Chin tucks* (E-8).

3. *Scapula squeezes* (E-2).

4. *Anterior chest stretch* (E-1).

5. *Bridge* (E-15).

6. *Single knee to chest into hamstring stretch* (E-16).

7. Hip flexor stretch. If the *psoas stretch* (E-21) is too challenging, you can perform the stretch lying down.

   a. To lengthen the muscles on the front of your thigh/hip, please do this stretch lying in bed. You will lie close to the edge of the bed and allow the leg closest to the edge to drop over the side while you bring the other leg up to your chest, using your arms to hug the leg. The leg that is off the bed hopefully has room to dangle and stretch. You can also try bending this knee to deepen the stretch.

8. Glute strengthening with *4-way hip* (E-20).

9. *Prone scapular squeeze into locust pose* (E-3).

10. *Quad stretch* (E-23).

11. *Deadlift* (E-26).

12. Standing posture/tadasana.

    a. Return to good posture.

    b. This isn't even a stretch, but a reminder to bring your body back to good posture. Bring back both hands to your low back (palms facing back) and rest them against the low back. Take deep, slow breaths while you hold the position for thirty seconds.

CHAPTER 14

MINDFULNESS MAGIC

"A healthy outside starts from the inside."
—Robert Urich

Anyone who has suffered from pain for extended periods will understand the deep emotional impact it has. You may feel depressed from being in constant pain, or anxious about when the next episode will hit. Maybe you are unable to concentrate or care for your children or ailing parents. Maybe you experienced loss of your job, leading to financial strain. You may even experience the feeling that getting out of bed to do your daily activities is physically impossible.

Pain and depression, as well as pain and anxiety, share similar biological pathways and neurotransmitters (chemicals) in the brain. Due to this, they often coexist, and conventional pain treatments are also antianxiety and antidepressant medications.

PAIN, DEPRESSION, AND ANXIETY

I first began doing research into the prevalence of pain in depressed individuals back in 2004. Since then, hundreds of studies have come out showing a significant relationship between depression and pain.

And the more severe a patient's pain is, the more severe their depression or anxiety may be.[1]

Research has shown that chronic pain affects the structure and functioning of the brain. In fact, many of the brain changes that take place during chronic pain also take place with depression and other mood disorders.

Compared to those without pain, chronic pain patients are shown to have between five percent and eleven percent less volume in the neocortex, the part of the brain responsible for higher functions such as rational thought, language, spatial reasoning, motor control, and sensory perception. This is similar to a ten- to twenty-year accelerated brain loss pattern.[2,3]

As we saw in Chapter 5, trauma and stress can not only trigger brain inflammation but also trigger physical symptoms such as Mind-Body Pain Syndrome.

Due to the profound impact of the mind on our body, it is critical you learn to turn off your fight-or-flight response, or your sympathetic autonomic nervous system (SNS). Luckily, it will still be there when you need it, jumping into action to help you run away from an attacker or ride a rollercoaster, but it is imperative to learn to come back to a state of balance in between the periods of time that your SNS is needed. Learning to do this will help you break your pain cycle.

This chapter will teach you how to use your brain to be its own pharmacy.

WHAT IS MINDFULNESS?

"Do not dwell in the past, do not dream of the future.
Concentrate the mind on the present moment."
—Buddha

Mindfulness has been recommended as a tool for chronic pain for thousands of years, although recently it has picked up mainstream attention. Ages ago, the Buddha taught his monks mindfulness as a means to overcome "sorrow and distress," as well as "for the disappearance of pain and sadness."[4]

Mindfulness is a state of awareness with one's own body. This awareness leads to you being present in any given moment. While practicing it, feelings, thoughts, and experiences come into awareness by teaching you to hold your attention on one given object or activity. This can be practiced while breathing, walking, sitting, or eating.

Part of the practice involves returning your thoughts to your body as well as to your breath. This requires letting go of other thoughts, worries, or past traumatic experiences that may creep into your mind. It even involves focusing on an unpleasant physical sensation your body may be experiencing at that time.

Some people with pain wonder how mindfulness will help them, when they feel all they are doing is focusing their thoughts on their physical pain. But surprisingly, even focusing just on one's physical symptoms improves overall pain levels because it removes other thoughts and emotions that often arise in conjunction with an episode of pain.

As people suffer from chronic pain, there is considerable focus on the physical aspect. What is often overlooked is the profound distress associated with living in pain. As we learned about in our mind-body chapters, many suffering from chronic pain have also suffered from emotional traumas, such as physical, mental, or sexual abuse. Others have suffered from other traumas, such as loss of their job, financial struggles, or relationship issues. These traumas are not physical but continuously injure your body. Mindfulness can negate that process.

By practicing mindfulness, we allow our bodies to heal and repair the damage done by these negative thoughts by regenerating and cultivating our parasympathetic pathways.[5,6,7,8]

HOW TO ACHIEVE MINDFULNESS

The first step is to begin with self-awareness. It is important to begin to pay attention to your needs, desires, emotions, and reactions to different situations. You need to learn to read your own internal cues so you can understand how your body is processing situations and expressing responses. Once you become aware of your emotional and physical state, you can begin to fine-tune your body to respond in a specific way.

It is important to learn your emotional and physical triggers and responses because they may differ from situation to situation. For example, on one day you may find yourself very anxious, which may trigger a headache or bout of back pain. And on another day, you may find yourself having severe hip pain, which may lead you to grow frustrated and respond with anger. By learning these cues and responses, we can make a conscious choice to overcome them and change our response, thereby mitigating all the negative chemical responses that follow.

This is where mindfulness practice comes into play. In this chapter, I am going to teach you to anchor yourself in the present moment, enabling you to increase self-awareness about your body.

The first thing is to set an intention for your mindfulness practice. What would you like to achieve? Do you want to improve your pain or manage day-to-day stress?

It is important to remember that this takes practice to truly reap the benefits. The wonderful part is it takes very little time. You only need to spend five minutes a day meditating or being mindful. This chapter will teach you how, and you can begin to incorporate this into your daily life.

STEP 1. REFLECTION

Go somewhere quiet. Sit or lie down in a comfortable, pain-free position. How do you feel? Are you sad, angry, anxious? If you are experiencing negative emotions, take a few deep diaphragmatic breaths. As you breathe, focus on what may be causing your negative thoughts. Bring yourself into the present moment. Focus on your belly moving as you breathe, the temperature of the room, and how each part of your body feels. Move from head to toe and think about how each part of your body feels at that moment. If you find yourself at a painful part of your body, stay there and take a few extra deep breaths. Then move on to the next body part.

Once you have completed this exercise, I want you to think about recent situations in your life. Think about experiences you have had in the last two days. Think about both positive and negative experiences. What was challenging about the negative experiences? How did they make you feel? Is there anything you would change about how you reacted? Is there any way you can change how you processed that situation to think about it in a less negative way? Think about your current relationships. Are any currently causing you stress?

Remember to do this often, particularly after you have a bad day or are in a bad mood. Practicing self-awareness about your feelings can improve your physical and mental health.

STEP 2. BREATHING

Diaphragmatic breathing is my favorite treatment for stress and anxiety. It is absolutely free and can be done anywhere! It can be helpful to process negative emotions and immediately relax your body's fight-or-flight response.[9]

Place your hand on your chest and another on your abdomen. Your abdomen should move, while your upper hand should not move much. Dr. Weil's 4–7–8 breath is an excellent way to return your body to a state of relaxation. Take a deep breath while counting to four, then hold the breath for seven counts, and exhale slowly through your nose for a count of eight.

Try to do this for five minutes each day before bedtime. I would also encourage you to do it as one to two breaths throughout your day, particularly when feeling anxious or feeling pain.

STEP 3. GUIDED IMAGERY

Think of a place that is relaxing and peaceful. Maybe it isn't a place you have visited but a place you have seen in photos. For some, it may be a white sandy beach with blue waves crashing in the background. For others, it may be in a cabin in the mountains. Wherever your peaceful setting is, I want you to find a quiet place to sit or lie down, close your eyes, and travel there.

Imagery is a type of meditation and requires practice. Studies have shown that by imagining an experience, you can generate the same physiological responses and emotions as if you were actually there.[10] With practice, you can do this on a regular basis for no cost at all.

Some scientists are studying virtual reality as treatments for a variety of conditions like anxiety and PTSD, and show early promising results.[11]

If you can harness your imagination and learn to truly immerse yourself in the scene, you can learn to do this on your own.

1. First choose your destination. Close your eyes and take yourself there mentally. Try to think of vivid details. What do you see around you? What temperature is it? What are you wearing? What sounds do you hear? If you reached out and touched something, what would it feel like?

2. Set a timer for five to ten minutes. You can do this for up to thirty minutes if you like.

3. If this is difficult for you, I recommend finding an audio guided imagery exercise.

STEP 4. MINDFUL EATING

Mindful eating is also a practice that needs to be learned. This is yet another way you can gain a deeper understanding of your mind and body. It refers to a philosophy of being attuned to your mind and its relationship with food. To begin you need to look at eating in a different light. Try to become aware of the reasons behind your hunger and the way you eat. Are certain emotions involved? Does food tie into your tradition? Do you eat based on your schedule—for example, eating on the go or in the car, no time to cook or eat healthily? Does your family have difficulty with access to food?

Being aware of our relationship to food is important for all of us, but particularly for people who have suffered from overeating, undereating, or other eating disorders. If you fall under this category, I strongly encourage you to seek professional guidance and utilize this tool as part of that therapy.

In the practice of mindful eating, it is important to listen to how your body feels. Allow yourself to eat without judgment. I don't expect you to eat mindfully all the time, but it is important to do this when possible. Again, it is a practice that must be learned. It may even take months until mindful eating is a natural part of your day.

TIPS FOR MINDFUL EATING

1. Prepare your meals. To truly learn to mindfully eat, I encourage you to cook for yourself. The first step in this process is to pay attention as you prepare food. Take in the sight of the food, the textures of how it feels, and the smells. If you are eating take-out or at a restaurant, try to pay attention to the smell and feel of the food.

2. Try to eat before you are starving. It will be difficult to mindfully eat if you are really hungry.

3. Go gadget-free. During mealtime, put your phone away. It is time to focus on food.

4. Be grateful. Before eating, take a moment to express gratitude for having the opportunity to eat the meal in front of you. If you have children who are picky eaters, this can be a good opportunity to instill gratitude in them as well.

5. Do not pay attention to diet or calories. This is about learning to connect with the food you eat.

6. Take small bites.

7. Chew slowly. This is a huge part of why American society is not eating mindfully on a regular basis and why we tend to overeat. I want you to chew until you can taste each part of the food. This may take ten to thirty chews per bite of food, depending on the food. As you chew, try to identify each of the ingredients and spices in each bite.

8. Minimize conversation. Try to spend the first five to ten minutes of your meal eating in this fashion and minimizing conversation, so you can pay attention to the flavors, textures, and smells.

STEP 5. MINDFUL MOVEMENT

Yoga, qi gong, and tai chi are excellent structured mindful movement practices. If you are able, I strongly encourage you to try these.

For those who would like a gentler introduction to mindful movement, you can try to incorporate a mindful walking practice.

TIPS FOR MINDFUL WALKING

1. Before you begin walking, pause. Become aware of your body and how it feels. Where has your weight settled, in your heels, or in the front part of your feet? Pay attention to your leg muscles that are holding you upright. Do they feel tight? Bend your knees slightly and see how that shifts your weight.

2. Begin to walk slowly, keeping your knees slightly bent. Pay attention to how your foot strikes the floor as you take each stride.

3. Continue to walk slowly, feeling the movement of your feet and how your body follows.

4. Take deep breaths as you walk, staying aware of the motion of your feet and body.

STEP 6. MEDITATION PRACTICE

I have had many patients tell me they tried meditation a couple times and failed. Or that as they meditate, their mind races, and therefore it did not work for them.

Our lives are very stressful. We are constantly on the move or plugged into our devices. Meditation is a time to restore your mind and body. Harnessing the beneficial aspects of meditation will allow you to reduce the negative physical effects of stress.

The health benefits of meditation are pretty outstanding. It reduces pain, anxiety, and depression and improves the immune system response.[12] Another thing to bear in mind is meditation improves productivity and mood, so for those who feel they cannot carve out the time for it, realize that it may actually make you focus and work more effectively.

From a physiological standpoint, meditation, which has been practiced around the world for thousands of years, can change your blood pressure, breathing patterns, and cortisol response.[13]

STEPS TO MEDITATE

1. Set aside five minutes a day. I recommend either right when you wake up or right before bed. To remind yourself, you can either have a meditation calendar or set a reminder on your phone. The best time to do this is after you have set aside your electronics for the evening or immediately before going to sleep.

2. Get comfortable, but you do not need to be in a special place for this.

3. Start with your diaphragmatic breathing.

4. Pay attention to the room you are in—take in the smells, listen to the sounds, and feel the temperature.

5. If you feel your mind wandering, come back to focusing on your breathing.

6. Scan your body from head to toe. Feel which areas are tense and which are relaxed.

7. If you find it difficult to stay in the present moment, you can do a guided imagery exercise and take yourself to a different place, where you can focus on experiencing the details of that environment.

8. Enjoy the silence and keep your mind on the present breath.

STEP 7. GRATITUDE JOURNALING

This is a beneficial exercise to bring you to a state of wellness. Please see Chapter 6 for details and instructions on how to do this.

STEP 8. FORGIVENESS

Events that have upset us affect our lives, some more deeply than others. And it is important that we grow from these situations so we do not repeat them. However, it is important also to remember that forgiveness is a huge part of recovering from those situations.

Forgiveness allows you to keep moving forward, whereas if you are stuck in an angry state, your body is holding onto those negative emotions and disabling your ability to heal. More than likely, the situation or person you are angry with has changed. Either the situation is over and will not repeat itself, or the person has changed. And if they have not, your ability to confront the issue either directly with them or internally within yourself, coupled with your ability to forgive, helps to get rid of that negative energy in your brain.

Holding on to anger does not change that the situation happened or change the individual that caused it—it only damages you. Learn to forgive and move on, even if you never forget. In Chapter 6, we have exercises on writing letters of forgiveness that may help.

MINDFULNESS-BASED STRESS REDUCTION (MBSR)

Mindfulness-based stress reduction is a program designed for patients with severe chronic pain to use mindfulness to decrease pain levels. The MSBR curriculum typically begins and ends with a body scan, or a meditation sequentially on each part of the body in the present state. This allows you to become aware of your breathing and aware of what parts of your body are in pain and how they relate to one another.

Patients often ask me how focusing on the painful body part is helpful, but over time it helps to correct avoidant behavior patterns that develop due to our anticipation of pain in a particular body part.

You can check out the Progressive Muscle Relaxation exercise in Chapter 6 for an introduction to sequential meditation.

Multiple studies have shown MBSR courses provide long-term pain relief for rheumatoid arthritis, back pain, fibromyalgia, and multiple other chronic pain diagnoses.[14,15,16,17]

An excellent free online six-week MBSR course can be found here: https://palousemindfulness.com/. You can also check out the Resources section or find an in-person course near you.

CONCLUSION

I see many patients, and was guilty of this myself, who turn to television, a glass of wine, or other unhealthy activities to combat stress. Restorative activities, such as those described in this chapter (meditation, mindfulness, journaling, diaphragmatic breathing, guided imagery) are extremely important science-backed ways to truly heal and promote wellness.

Taking even a few minutes each day to do these restorative activities can lead to lasting improvements in your overall health and well-being. It can reduce pain, improve sleep, improve resiliency, increase your immune system, balance hormones, and decrease anxiety.

CHAPTER 15

SLEEP SOUNDLY

"Sleep is the best meditation."
—Dalai Lama

WHY SLEEP IS IMPORTANT

Believe it or not, treating sleep is the key to treating most chronic pain disorders. Anxiety, depression, and chronic pain can cause difficulty sleeping, and poor sleep worsens these conditions.[1,2,3] Optimizing sleep will not only improve these conditions, but also it will reduce the brain fog and fatigue that often coexist with pain.

RULE OUT A SLEEP DISORDER

The first step is to rule out a sleep disorder. Visit www.sleepapnea.org or check the CDC website for the Epworth Sleepiness Scale Quiz.

If you are at high risk per the questionnaire, discuss the results with your doctor. A common cause of daytime fatigue and fogginess is undiagnosed sleep apnea. You should visit www.stopbang.ca to take the STOP-BANG risk questionnaire. If you are either intermediate or high risk, talk with your doctor about getting a sleep study. Your sleep level and overall health will drastically improve with appropriate treatment.

For those who don't have insurance coverage for a sleep study, home sleep studies cost around $200–$300 versus an overnight stay of about $1,000. Usually both are covered by insurance. If you choose to purchase one to do at home, I cannot guarantee its validity.

Treatment for obstructive sleep apnea varies based on the stage. It may be weight loss, adjusted sleep positions, dental devices, or a CPAP machine.

RESTLESS LEG SYNDROME

Reports show 50 to 60 percent of people suffer from nighttime painful leg cramping that can be very disruptive to sleep. There could be multiple causes, making it challenging to treat. Some labs that should be checked are CBC and ferritin to monitor iron, B_{12} levels, and magnesium levels. There is some evidence that magnesium supplements and vitamin B_{12} supplementation can help. You can discuss these with your doctor.

I recommend getting regular exercise in the daytime, staying hydrated by drinking plenty of water throughout the day, stretching before bed, and either taking a warm bath or using a heating pad on your calves before bedtime.

A fifteen-minute stretching sequence focusing on your legs and calf muscles is key before bed.

Restless leg syndrome is also commonly seen in patients with small intestinal bacterial overgrowth (SIBO), so restoring microbial gut balance may help alleviate symptoms.

If the above methods fail, some prescription therapies that can help reduce symptoms include gabapentin, pregabalin, and Metanx (a prescription vitamin).

REVIEW YOUR LIST OF MEDICATIONS

Thoroughly check your medication list with your doctor to make sure you are taking medications at the right time and that none cause insomnia. Interestingly, I often see patients using opioids or benzodiazepines like Ativan to help them sleep. They typically aid in helping you fall asleep but reduce your time spent in deep sleep. These medications can actually promote fatigue in the long run.[4] If you are on benzodiazepines, talk to your doctor about when to take them for anxiety, and utilize other methods to aid in sleep. If you are planning to wean off of these medications, discuss the safest way to do so with your doctor.

Some other medications that interfere with sleep include:

- Cold medications

- Asthma medications

- Blood pressure medications

- Thyroid medications

- Antidepressants

- Stimulants like Adderall or Ritalin

- Some pain medications (morphine, methadone)

If you take any of these and have difficulty sleeping, discuss alternatives with your doctor.

NOTE ON SLEEP TRACKING APPS

There are apps that can track sleep quality, but it is difficult to say whether those are accurate or helpful. In fact, research has found sleep-tracking technology can actually worsen sleep quality as people become obsessed with tracking sleep quality, and this increases their insomnia. Instead of tracking, I suggest following the suggestions in this chapter. With higher quality sleep, you will feel better the next day. That's all the tracking you need.

IMPROVE SLEEP HYGIENE

1. Go outside for a morning stroll. Seeing daylight in the morning increases your natural levels of melatonin so your body knows when it is daytime and when it is nighttime.

2. Decrease exposure to blue light. Blue light inhibits melatonin and stimulates the production of cortisol, the stress hormone. Increased exposure via screens or the sun can shorten sleep time and quality. Solution: Wear blue light blocking glasses. These can help some headache sufferers during the day as well if you are using a screen a lot. But I recommend blocking blue light by wearing these glasses for three hours before bed and even possibly throughout the night, depending on your exposure levels. If possible, it is helpful to keep all electronic devices away from you. However, for many this isn't possible, so the blue light glasses can be helpful. You can buy some designed for sleep on Amazon for $10–$30, and you can also have a blue light blocker added to your lenses for pretty affordable prices online. You should also set your phone to night mode each evening around two hours before your bedtime until around 7:00 a.m. This ensures your phone displays less blue light during those hours.

3. Choose the right sleeping equipment. We spend an exorbitant amount of time in our beds, so it is crucial to choose the ideal mattress, pillow, and sleeping position. Inadequate support in any of these areas will cause or worsen muscle tension and pain.

- **Pillow** – I personally prefer memory foam contour pillows, but pillows are a personal choice and sometimes require some trial and error. If you sleep on your back, choose a very thin pillow or the thinner side of a contour pillow. Your neck should feel neutral. If you sleep on your side, choose a pillow that allows your neck to be straight. I personally recommend the Milemont Memory Foam Pillow on Amazon or a Tempur-Pedic Contour Pillow that provides support for your neck and has two sides so you can find the ideal thickness to keep your neck neutral. You may be able to find a local mattress store with a sixty-day return policy. Amazon also has some quality options with thirty-day returns.

- **Mattress** – You need to sleep on a medium or firm mattress that supports your body. Very soft mattresses are usually bad for your back. The ideal mattress allows your hips and shoulders to remain aligned with your spine when sleeping on your side. You need to choose firmness based on your body weight. Mattress firmness is particularly important for side sleepers. Your hips and shoulders must sink a little so that your spine remains neutral. The heavier you are, the firmer your mattress needs to be to provide the right support. You should always try out your mattress and find a store that allows you to return after thirty or sixty days. The longer the trial period, the better. And don't change your mattress and pillow at the same time because you will not be able to tell which is the source of increased pain.

- **Sleep position** – You spend six to eight hours in this position every night, so it is extremely important you are in a good position. When you're sleeping, your spine should be aligned from your tailbone to your head. If you sleep on your side, place a pillow between your knees to improve alignment and a contour pillow under your neck so your hips and spine are neutral. If you sleep on your back, place a pillow underneath your legs. If you shift positions, your pillow needs to shift with you. I do not recommend stomach sleeping.

4. Don't consume caffeine after lunchtime.

5. Don't consume alcohol for five hours before bedtime. It has a negative impact on sleep.[5]

6. Avoid large meals and large quantities of liquid two hours before bedtime.

7. Avoid intense exercise four hours before bedtime.

8. Two hours before bedtime, start dimming the lights. Remember to avoid blue light and minimize using your computer or watching television.

9. An hour before bed, write down a list of things you have to do or things you are anxious about. Place the list in a drawer next to your bed. This is so you know you won't forget them, but also to remind you not to worry about them for the rest of the night.

10. Take a warm bath or shower to ease any muscle aches and relax you. Consider using fragrant essential oils in your bath, like lavender or Epsom bath salts.

11. Wear comfortable, loose sleeping clothes.

12. If you are sensitive to noises, turn on white noise, or use earplugs.

13. Make sure the room is dark (use blackout curtains or an eye patch) and cool (around sixty-five to sixty-eight degrees). Minimize light in your bedroom from cell phones, laptops, windows, alarm clocks, TVs, and any other electronics.

14. If you are hungry before bed, eat a light snack, not a heavy meal.

15. If you are often wide awake in the middle of the night, try a light snack with protein and fat before bed to reduce nighttime cortisol spikes.

16. Consider using a weighted blanket, particularly if you suffer from anxiety.

If you implement all these techniques and still cannot sleep, some supplements and herbs can help with sleep but should always be discussed with your doctor. Some of these include melatonin, valerian root, and Rhodiola. If you have trouble falling asleep, consider melatonin (0.5–5 mg) thirty to sixty minutes before bedtime. If you have trouble staying asleep, try a time-release melatonin. If melatonin does not work, consider discussing this supplement blend for sleep, Best Rest Formula by Pure Encapsulations, with your doctor.

If these techniques do not work, I recommend discussing with your provider prescription options to improve sleep, such as neuropathic (nerve) medications, muscle relaxants, or certain antidepressants shown effective for pain and sleep. These work particularly well for those with chronic pain.

CHAPTER 16

TAME THE TOXINS

"If someone wishes for good health, one must first ask oneself if he is ready to do away with the reasons for his illness. Only then is it possible to help him."
—Hippocrates

We are surrounded by chemicals, and some degree of exposure is inevitable. Many believe this is why we are seeing escalating doses of chronic disease today that were nonexistent in our ancestors. The goal of this chapter is to educate you on where some of these toxins and chemicals are coming from, and provide steps you can take to protect yourself.

Environmental toxins have been shown to cause damage to our gut, nervous systems, and cognition. Nerve pain, headaches, and brain fog are just some of the symptoms that can improve with minimizing or removing toxins. As we learned in the central pain chapter (Chapter 7), toxins can be a hidden cause of mysterious pain symptoms.

Your goal is not to live an entirely toxin-free life. No one can physically do that. The goal is to reduce the overall toxin burden. Unfortunately, this chapter contains some alarming warnings, and some of these issues, like the food we eat or the water we drink, can seem so daunting that we might not know where to start. The point of this chapter is not to cause stress—in fact, that would be counter-productive. The aim is to point out potential factors that may be contributing to pain. Please note that some changes toward the positive are always better than none. If you are trying to add more fruits and vegetables to your diet but cannot afford organic foods, know that you are still doing good things for your body. Any amount of fruit and vegetables, organic or not, will be far more healing to your body than processed and packaged foods. However, I've included this section so that if you have the time and energy, you can fine-tune your diet and lifestyle even more by eliminating potentially harmful toxins that can create problems over time. Each section contains a "baby step" that you can try in order to move forward in that area.

If you are currently suffering from extreme anxiety or obsessive-compulsive disorders, you may want to hold off on reading or implementing this section until you have a good handle on the basic lifestyle changes in Chapters 10, 12, 13, 14, and 15.

You can take this questionnaire to give yourself an idea of your exposure. For each question, you should answer "often," "occasionally," "in the past," or "no." If you answer "often" to a section, this is something you should aim to address first. If you answer "occasionally," consider working on reducing this exposure as you are able.

HOME EXPOSURES

1. Do you live in an apartment or home built before 1978?

2. Do you live in a mobile home, boat, or RV?

3. Does your home contain new construction materials or furniture?

4. Does your home or workplace show signs of mold or water damage?

5. Are you exposed to conventional cleaning products, including air fresheners, scented candles, etc.?

6. Do you live or work near an industrial pollution source? Near a source with electromagnetic radiation, like a cell phone tower?

OUTDOOR EXPOSURES

1. Do you often visit parks or other outdoor areas that are likely treated with herbicides or pesticides? In public areas, there are often signs, plant flags, or even colored dye mixed in with the herbicides that indicate when an area has been treated with these chemicals. You can check your state's website for what their rules are.

2. Do you run or bike along busy streets with lots of traffic?

3. Are you exposed to toxic chemicals by activities you do (examples: gasoline, paint, adhesives, glues, etc.)?

PERSONAL EXPOSURES

1. Do you use a lot of scented lotions, products, shampoos, etc.? Are you sensitive to them?

2. Do you smoke, or are you exposed to secondhand smoke?

3. Do you have a history of substance abuse or use alcohol or recreational drugs?

4. Do you have silver fillings? Dental implants?

5. Do you have any artificial materials in your body like implants?

INDOOR AIR POLLUTANTS

Environmental toxins are everywhere. Many of us know very little about them and how they are impacting our health. Experts estimate we are currently exposed to over 80,000 chemicals, and each year that list grows.

Surprisingly, very few of these chemicals have been rigorously tested for their effects on our organ systems. Even so, it is important to look at these toxins as another source that may explain why we are experiencing higher levels of chronic disease than our ancestors. The Environmental Protection Agency (EPA) notes that indoor and outdoor air pollution can be associated with a number of health concerns, including heart attacks, bronchitis, asthma, and infections. In fact, the EPA estimates that we have worse air quality indoors than we do outdoors.

Although we do not definitively know that these chemicals are causing fatigue, headaches, and pain issues, there have been plenty of reports indicating that in certain individuals, they can. The list below reviews some harmful chemical sources.

1. Tobacco from cigarettes, as well as certain cooking appliances and fireplaces, can release harmful combustion byproducts such as carbon monoxide.

2. Cleaning supplies, paints, insecticides, and other commonly used products introduce many different chemicals, including volatile organic compounds, directly into the indoor air.

3. Scented candles and many air fresheners are another source of indoor pollution. They also don't remove bad odors; they just mask them with chemicals. EWG.org has studied air fresheners and found some contained as many as eighty-nine airborne contaminants, including acetaldehyde. The solution? Run a fan or open a window. Or use the filter mentioned in #5.

4. Buildings and building materials are also potential sources. Some buildings contain asbestos, radon, and mold. New

construction homes have a mixture of chemicals in them, including formaldehyde and VOCs (volatile organic compounds). These chemicals evaporate into the air from paint, sealants, flooring, and other building materials. These will continue to be released over the first few years of a new home and lead to pollutant levels that may be two to six times as much as outdoor pollution! Refer to #5.

5.   If you can afford it, an indoor HEPA filter is a great investment, particularly for those with indoor allergies. If not, try to spend time outdoors every day, and open windows to ventilate your homes, particularly after cleaning or using your fireplace.

BABY STEPS

Skip the scented candles and air fresheners altogether, and every day be sure to run a fan and open your windows.

FOOD POLLUTANTS

It is best to try to avoid pesticides, germicides, and fungicides. These can be found in food. Try to opt for organic produce when possible. I understand this is very costly, so I suggest visiting www.EWG.org and find their list for the Dirty Dozen (foods with the highest amount of pesticides) and the Clean Fifteen (lowest amount). Try to buy organic for the Dirty Dozen and save your money on the Clean Fifteen.

There is growing evidence on the relationship between exposure to pesticides and higher numbers of chronic diseases such as cancers, diabetes, birth defects, reproductive issues, and neurodegenerative disorders like Parkinson, Alzheimer's, and amyotrophic lateral sclerosis (ALS).[1] There is also possible evidence of a link between pesticides and other chronic diseases like asthma, chronic obstructive pulmonary disease (COPD), heart disease, chronic nerve pain disorders, autoimmune diseases like Lupus and rheumatoid arthritis, and chronic fatigue syndrome. Researchers suspect this is due to the pesticides causing an issue with cellular regulation.[2]

BABY STEPS

If cost is an issue, try to purchase organic for only the items on the Dirty Dozen, or spend a lot of time washing your produce prior to eating it. Better yet, grow your own herbs and produce!

CLEAN WATER

Even good-quality tap water may contain chloride, fluoride, and environmental pollutants like pesticides and other chemicals. Unfortunately, the quality of bottled water isn't always better because you are potentially exposing yourself to harmful plastic particles. Please also remember that we must think of the future of the Earth as well. The amount of trash we accumulate, not to mention the cost of bottled water, is plenty of reason to try to find a filtered option. Another concern is that sometimes bottled water can contain these same pollutants and chemicals. There is no guarantee of its purity. Investing in a good water filter is usually worthwhile.

Do your homework to find a good filter. The best thing to do is check out the EWG.org tap water source website. Type in your zip code and see what contaminants are in your drinking water.

Believe it or not, there are over three hundred contaminants in our tap water, and the EPA only looks for one hundred of them. There are individual labs that can go into this further.

For some of you, buying a home water filtration system is an option, but for others it may not be feasible. Luckily, there are some high-quality countertop water filters. Unfortunately, none of the high-quality options are particularly cheap.

The best-selling water pitchers, like Brita, actually do very little to remove the contaminants in tap water. They are primarily used to remove chlorine and make the water taste better. Unfortunately, they may leave behind toxic substances such as herbicides, pesticides, and lead.

Look for what contaminants are in your area's water to find the most cost-effective option for your household. The two best types of water filters are those with carbon filters and reverse osmosis filters. Some over-the-counter water filters that I think are worth the investment are the Big Berkey and AquaTru brands. Both are pricey at over $250, but they do a nice job and provide certifications on their websites. For those on a budget who still want to try to drink the cleanest water possible, you can search online for groups who have done third-party testing on much more affordable water pitchers to find a quality one. The EWG website has a section on water filters as well.

BABY STEPS

Check the EWG website for your area's water quality. If the water quality is poor and you cannot afford a water filter, you can check your local grocery store for water vending machines, which are usually very affordable. Be sure to check what type of filter the machine has.

ELECTROMAGNETIC STRESS

We are surrounded by electromagnetic stress throughout our day. We are constantly around devices such as cell phones, TVs, computers, and microwaves. There is some thought that an excess of these electromagnetic frequencies can cause issues like poor sleep, fatigue, and memory issues.

BABY STEPS

Sleep with your phone at least two to three feet away from your head. Try not to have a TV in your bedroom. Consider shutting off your Wi-Fi at night.

Try to avoid microwaving your food.

MOLD

One of the most underdiagnosed ties to nerve pain and Central Pain Syndrome is mold. Mold has become very widespread and can grow in your home without your knowledge.

To avoid mold, your home's humidity level should not exceed 50 percent. Some of the first symptoms of mold-induced illness are morning stiffness, brain fog, fatigue, sleep disturbances, digestive issues, headaches, and poor memory.

For basements or other damp areas of the home, use a dehumidifier to keep the area dry and discourage the growth of mold. For areas in your home with visible mold, consider calling a mold remediation specialist to assess the severity and determine what should be done. Be mindful that every home will have some level of mold in it, particularly in the basement, and not all mold needs to be removed extensively. These professional companies are extremely expensive and often provide quotes for levels of remediation that are above what you need. You can also refer to your state's health department for guidance. If you think you have been exposed to mold and that it is triggering symptoms, you can see a functional medicine practitioner who can work with you on treatment.

BABY STEPS

If you live in a home with a lot of mold and are unable to afford mold remediation, you can see if the mold is causing you problems by checking if your symptoms improve when you are away from home for seven to ten days. If they do, then you can pursue the options above.

PLASTICS

Plastic is everywhere. Unfortunately, that means phthalates are as well. Phthalates are cancer-causing and hormone-disrupting chemicals in plastic.

You may have heard the term BPA-free, but BPA-free plastic does not necessarily mean you are totally out of the woods. BPA is bisphenol A, and some research has linked it to fertility problems, heart disease, and impotence. It is typically taken out of all baby products and a lot of food storage plastics.

BPA has a similar structure to estrogen, and experts think that explains why it has some harmful hormonal effects. However, other experts say the levels in our plastics are low enough not to cause any issues. The jury is still out on this one, but it is still a good idea to avoid the "bad plastics" since hormones have been tied to chronic pain issues as we discussed in our central pain chapter.

The Society of the Plastics Industry (SPI) came up with a numbering system to classify plastics for recycling purposes. Every piece of plastic has a number on the bottom of it from 1 to 7. Plastics with the numbers 1, 2, 4, and 5 are safest. You should avoid plastics with numbers 3, 6, and 7. Plastics labeled 3 and 7 typically contain BPA.

Heat causes these chemicals to leach out of plastic, so do not microwave plastic. Foods can absorb chemicals released by plastic when it's heated in the microwave.

BABY STEPS

Try to use glass or steel water bottles and food storage containers when possible.

PERSONAL CARE PRODUCTS

Unfortunately, dozens of chemicals can be found in conventional shampoos, soaps, makeup, skincare products, cosmetics, lotions, and perfumes. These chemicals have been tied to cancer, diabetes, depression, and a whole host of inflammatory conditions that can be tied to chronic pain.

The studies are big and frightening when you dig through them. Not only does the United States allow thousands of chemicals in its skincare products that other countries like the United Kingdom have banned, but the risks of these chemicals are hardly minor.

If you visit the EWG Skin Deep website (https://www.ewg.org/skindeep/), you can type in a particular brand or product and find its safety ratings. The safest of them all will have an EWG verified green symbol, indicating that the product is free of a long list of harmful chemicals.

BABY STEPS

Try to replace only the items that you are using frequently and that have the potential to be absorbed, such as your body wash or deodorant. There is no need to replace every single item in your bathroom.

SUMMARY POINTS

The aim of this chapter was to educate, not frighten you. I apologize if I did the latter. It may seem like an impossible task to replace all toxins in your home with safer products. I do not expect you to do that, nor have I. Your goal should be to do the best you can. Start with baby steps. Take your time, and remember to always be kind to yourself.

Some helpful resources are www.ewg.org and the book *Non-Toxic: Guide to Living Healthy in a Chemical World* by Aly Cohen.

CHAPTER 17

YOUR PAIN TREATMENT TOOLBOX

George was a fifty-six-year-old gentleman who had undergone back surgery for excruciating pain in his low back. Unfortunately, he woke up from the surgery with the exact same pain he had before the surgery. The surgeon had referred him to my clinic when he was still experiencing pain and requiring narcotics two months after the surgery. The surgeon said, "He probably needs an epidural injection."

I asked George what types of treatments he had done prior to surgery, whether he had tried an epidural injection before, or even done any physical therapy. He looked at me and said that no one ever mentioned physical therapy or any injections. I asked if he had tried massage or chiropractic care, and he stated that with his insurance (he was on public aid) and financial status, that was impossible. I did a physical exam, took a thorough history, and told him that I thought his pain was primarily muscular.

I instructed him to begin physical therapy and told him that he would benefit from a heating pad, exercise, and stretching. He was still skeptical that the pain was just muscular since he attributed his pain to disc bulges previously seen on his MRI. We decided to proceed with ultrasound-guided trigger point injections into his back muscles. I only needed to do four areas. These injections were done with numbing medicine (local anesthetic) so we could see relief right away if we had numbed the right spot. When I went to check on him five minutes after the procedure, he stood up and said, "I have no pain. I can't believe it. For the first time in two years, I have no pain. What does that mean?" I said, "Well, it means we found our source."

At the six-week follow-up visit, he had not yet started any sort of exercise program and had not even purchased a heating pad due to cost. Consequently, the pain had returned in a month. Not only did his financial hardship limit his ability to get chiropractic care and massage therapy, but we were also denied approval for additional trigger point injections, which he so desperately wanted. There was a nine-week wait for physical therapy at the university physical therapy clinic, the only place he could afford to travel to that took his insurance. Every other place in the city that took public aid required him to travel there by bus, and he could not afford the bus fare. He was in tears.

With some counseling and creativity, I was able to design a routine that he could afford. I gave him instructions to make his own heating pad and use a tennis ball to do myofascial release. We added ergonomic changes and some home exercises, and after three and a half months of following this program, his pain entirely resolved and never returned.

As we saw in Chapter 12, everything you do day to day impacts not only your current pain status but also future pain issues. Everything from what pillow you are using and what shoes you're wearing to how you text and even how you breathe impacts whether you'll be suffering from pain in five to ten years.

It is important to be proactive and to work to preserve your current body. You only have one for this whole life, after all. It is important that when you begin to notice pain in a given area, you take action so the pain cycle cannot begin.

This chapter will talk about my favorite products to self-manage pain and DIY hacks for those who can't afford some of these items but still need relief. As always with this book, the key is self-maintenance. When something is sore for more than a few days, don't ignore it.

FOOTWEAR

Supportive footwear is key. See Chapter 12.

SEAT CUSHIONS

These can be enormously helpful for those suffering from low back pain, sciatica, hip pain, buttock pain, and sacroiliac joint issues. You can use this while driving, traveling in a plane, or sitting at home or work.

Recommended product: Everlasting Comfort has an excellent one (Everlasting Comfort Seat) for $32 on Amazon.

DIY: Try to sit in a supportive seat as much as possible (your dining room chair vs. your couch).

BACK (LUMBAR) SUPPORT CUSHION

These are really important to prevent low back discomfort, particularly if sitting in one spot for over twenty minutes.

Recommended product: The Original McKenzie Inflatable Lumbar Support Pillow because it can be adjusted.

DIY: A rolled-up towel or small pillow placed in the curve of your low back.

SELF-MYOFASCIAL TOOLS

Unsticking your fascia is a huge component in managing chronic pain, particularly for those suffering from centralized pain or fibromyalgia-type pain. In the Resources, I explain how to find a myofascial release therapist trained in either the Barnes' therapy or rolfing (another technique of massage), but you can also begin to practice self-myofascial release at home (see suggestions below). You can check with your insurance carrier, as myofascial release massage may be covered with a doctor's prescription.

Fascia is a type of connective tissue surrounding your muscles, nerves, and blood vessels.[1] Areas of tension in the fascia that are due to poor body mechanics or injury can lead to severe pain. Soft tissue mobilization using these tools can increase flexibility, improve blood flow, and decrease recovery time after an injury.[2,3]

It is important to remember that tightness in one area, such as the hamstring, can actually cause pain in another area (the low back).

It is best to do self-myofascial release (SMFR) after you exercise, not before, about two to three times a week.

You can learn how to do self-myofascial release via the MELT method by Sue Hitzmann or by reading *Myofascial Stretching: A Guide to Self-Treatment* by Jill Stedronsky and Brenda Pardy.

On www.drdecaria.com, there are instructions on how to do SMFR with a tennis ball, but you can also use some of my favorite myofascial tools listed here. I will also add some DIY options.

Recommended product: 321 Strong Foam Roller

DIY: Make one with one-inch PVC pipe inside of a 24 inch foam noodle.

Recommended product: Thera cane

Unfortunately, no simple DIY recommendations for this one.

Recommended product: OPTP Stretching Strap to help stretch your hamstrings

DIY: Dog leash or two neckties tied together

Recommended product: The Idson Muscle Roller Stick. This is great to use on thighs, hamstrings, calves, and IT band.

DIY: Rolling pin

Recommended product: Spoiled Hippo massage trigger point ball.

DIY: Tennis ball. You can also place two tennis balls in a tube sock, tie the sock, and roll out larger areas like your back or neck muscles against a wall.

BALANCE BOARD

If you are in relatively good shape, using a balance board for five minutes a day is an excellent way to keep your stability muscles working and strong.

Recommended product: The <u>Strongtec Professional Wooden Balance Board</u>.

DIY: Using a round piece of wood, friction tape, and a wooden pine ball top and screws, you can make one yourself.

Note: If you have balance issues, weakness, or are deconditioned and do not regularly exercise, a balance board is not for you.

BACK BRACE

Back braces should only be used when indicated by your doctor or physical therapist. They are typically used after you have surgery or if you have had a vertebral fracture. Long-term use of back braces for non-traumatic low back pain or back pain caused by muscle issues (like the majority of chronic back pain) can create more damage. This is because it weakens your muscles over time since they are not being used while in the brace.

SUPPORT BELTS DURING PREGNANCY

I would consult with your obstetrician or a physical therapist on this, but support belts are incredibly beneficial when used properly during pregnancy to help avoid low back strain. There are different ones to use for different stages of pregnancy. I used all of them at various points. Support pillows at night for proper sleep positioning are also key. There are many designed for the different stages of pregnancy.

SACROILIAC (SI) JOINT BELTS

For those suffering from sacroiliac joint pain, which is an alarming number of people, SI joint belts can be super helpful. There's a learning curve with these, so I do recommend bringing this up with your physical therapist or pain physician to see if it's a good choice and having them show you exactly how to wear it.

Recommended product: The SI-LOC belt, which comes in different sizes based on your waist.

DIY: You can wear a tight leather belt, low on your hips over the bony protuberances in your low back (the posterior superior iliac spine). If you look at the SI-LOC listing on Amazon it shows you where it should be worn.

TAPING

If you've ever done physical therapy, particularly for an issue such as tendinitis, you may have been taped by your physical therapist. Or maybe you've seen professional sports players with colored tape on their arms or legs. Patients often report that this provides excellent relief of their pain. Good news—with instruction—you can learn to tape areas of pain yourself. Unlike the issue with back braces, kinesiology tape works by supporting your muscles but still allowing you to use them.

Kinesiology tape is around $8–$16 per roll and available online. Once applied, it can be worn for several days, as it is waterproof and holds up nicely.

The theory behind this flexible, elastic tape (which is different from other cloth tapes) is that the elastic core fibers in the tape, when applied correctly, reduce pressure to the tissue, which can help to reduce pain. It also works to support your muscles and keep them neutral, so you do not overcontract or overextend them.

Taping can be used to stabilize muscles, joints, and tendons that have been strained or are aching. It can also remind you to remain in good posture. Visit this website for more specifics on how to apply it and for what conditions: https://www.kttape.com/how-to-apply-kt-tape.

Ideally, your physical therapist can teach you how to use it, and then you can do it at home, because there is a learning curve in how to do this properly.

As with anything, if it hurts after you put it on, something's wrong, and you should remove it.

TENS UNIT

TENS units are small devices that can be used to help chronic pain. They work by using adhesive pads attached to electrodes that deliver small electrical impulses. The theory behind a TENS unit is that these signals flood the nervous system and reduce its ability to transmit pain signals to our brain and spinal cord. Some believe it produces natural pain relievers or endorphins, although this has not been scientifically proven.

They are typically worn for fifteen- to forty-minute sessions once to twice daily. Many are discrete and have batteries, so they can be worn even when out and about. They are safe, non-invasive options. However, there are a few negatives. Here is a list of some of the drawbacks: there is limited research so far, the cost of adhesive pads can add up, you can't use if you have adhesive allergies, and some patients find the tingling, electrical sensation actually painful. (I find that this is often the case with my central pain patients who have sensitivity to touch.) It is important not to use this over your face or neck, or near any blood vessels. You also cannot use it if you have a pacemaker or metal implants, are pregnant, or have epilepsy or heart problems.

However, many of my patients with back pain and hip pain do find relief with their TENS units.

You can purchase one by TENS 7000 on Amazon for under $30, or you can try to have your doctor prescribe one through your insurance (like the Zynex device, which has some additional capabilities). I personally prefer the Zynex or other prescription TENS units, although the Amazon one is a decent option as well.

HEATING PAD

Superficial heat in the form of a heat wrap has been shown to moderately improve acute low back pain. When combined with exercise, it also appears to improve pain and function in patients with acute low back pain more than exercise alone.[4]

Heat is typically best for muscle pain. If you go back to Chapters 3 and 4, there is more detail on how to tell if it is a muscle, joint, or tendon that is bothering you. You can pick up a heating pad from your local pharmacy or online.

DIY HEATING PAD

You can make a reusable heating pad out of an old, clean tube sock. Take a large sock and fill it three-quarters full with uncooked rice. Then tie or sew it shut and heat in the microwave for one minute. Always test a heating pad on the inside of the arm before applying it to the affected area. If you freeze the sock, you can use it as an ice pack.

ICE PACK

An ice pack can cost anywhere from $8–$20. If you have a larger area you want to ice, like your hip, the larger ones are closer to $15.

Recommended product: I recommend this large Comfort Gel Pack because you can use it as a hot or cold pack on your hip or across your low back.

DIY: Bag of frozen peas or the tube sock mentioned above.

SQUATTY POTTY OR RESTROOM STOOL

Use one of these! If you have no bowel issues or back issues, you likely have never paid attention to the position in which you use the restroom. But I have often heard patients say their pain is aggravated while using the restroom.

Many people in Asia and Africa have routinely squatted while using the restroom, but in Western societies we sit on the toilet. The issue with sitting is that it keeps the kink in your lower bowel. What does that mean? You have to work harder to push out the stool. When you squat, and bend your hips and knees, you straighten out your colon, relax your puborectalis muscle, and the stool can be passed easily with less straining.

Recommended product: The Squatty Potty ® can be purchased online.

DIY: You can also simply bend your hips and bring your knees up or be creative and use a stool or other objects to rest your feet on. Ideally you want your feet resting on something at least seven inches off the ground.

CRANIOSACRAL POSITIONING DEVICE

These positioning devices can help with cervical/neck headaches, head/neck muscle tension, or migraine/occipital headaches. You can find an excellent one at www.craniocradle.com.

INFRARED SAUNAS

Many other countries use infrared saunas for therapy. You can purchase one for home use or find a place that provides affordable sessions. There are studies supporting the use of infrared sauna therapy for back pain, fatigue, fibromyalgia, and muscle pain.[5,6]

TOPICAL TREATMENTS

Medications all carry significant risks. If you read through the inserts of the medications you pick up or purchase over the counter, you've probably noticed that the side effects are frightening. Did you know Tylenol can cause liver disease and death?

With any of these, please check ingredients and consult your doctor to make sure you aren't allergic to anything and that it won't interact with your current medications. Even topical creams and patches lead to some absorption of the product into your bloodstream.

These primarily provide temporary relief and are not a long-term fix. But temporary relief may be really helpful for you as you try to address the root cause of pain with this book.

In my quest to find relief, I think I have tried at least fifty different topical products. My favorite over-the-counter topical rubs and patches, in no particular order, are Biofreeze roll-on or topical gel, doTERRA Deep Blue Rub, Salonpas patches, Golden Sunshine Herbal Pain Patch, Arnicare cream, and Voltaren (diclofenac sodium 1%) gel. Voltaren is an NSAID anti-inflammatory gel usually used for knee arthritis—ask your doctor if on blood thinners or taking other anti-inflammatories.

CBD (CANNABIDIOL)

Unless you have been living under a rock, you have probably heard of CBD. It seems lately you can get it anywhere, from a department store to a smoothie shop. Cannabidiol (CBD) oils are low tetrahydrocannabinol (THC) products derived from the *Cannabis sativa* plant. Patients report relief for a variety of conditions, particularly pain, without the intoxicating adverse effects of marijuana/cannabis. It comes in a variety of forms, including topical patches, creams, and oral oils.

In June 2018, the first CBD-based drug, Epidiolex, was approved by the U.S. Food and Drug Administration for the treatment of severe epilepsy. Despite the fact that there are very few large well-designed trials, there is a growing body of clinical evidence to support the use of CBD for a number of conditions, such as arthritis, nerve pain, cancer pain, anxiety, insomnia, and opioid addiction.[7,8,9,10,11]

However, one must be very careful in choosing CBD products because there is little to no regulation. Studies have found inaccurate labeling of products and even the possibility of harmful contaminants. I recommend discussing brands with your healthcare provider to find those that are batch tested, are sourced in the U.S., and use good manufacturing practices.

FINAL THOUGHTS:
STAYING ON TRACK

"Nothing is impossible. The word itself says I'm possible."
—Audrey Hepburn

For many who read this book, you may feel like this is far too much to accomplish. You may feel like there is no way you can implement this program while being in so much pain you are unable to move. Changing one's lifestyle is one of the most challenging tasks we can do and why we have had so much difficulty overcoming this battle with chronic pain. Since the healthcare system is designed to mask symptoms with a pill or surgery, many of us have learned to face pain with the same attitude. I hope through reading this book, you have realized that that system is broken. You will not be able to truly heal unless you decide it's time to make a change.

I also completely understand that you are overwhelmed, exhausted, busy working, and worrying about being a burden, and you may even be a caregiver. I understand that for some, getting out of bed and brushing your teeth feels impossible. The thought of doing an entirely new diet, journaling, exercising, and practicing mindfulness seems insurmountable.

I also understand that implementing many of the aspects of Part 2 in this book may be costly, time-consuming, and for some of you, out of reach.

If you are anything like me, when you have a ton of stuff you want to do, it is easy to get overwhelmed and have no idea where to start. To combat that feeling, I have summarized the nuts and bolts of my recommendations in the following list. Choose where to start, and gradually work your way through the list.

QUICK GUIDE ON HOW TO LIVE WELL IN AN UNWELL WORLD

1. Use the Pain Syndrome Questionnaire to determine your pain type and what therapies/providers you need to seek out to break your cycle.

2. Go outside. For those in colder climates, get a happy light therapy lamp like the one by Miroco to use in winter (use for twenty minutes every morning).

3. Drink clean water.

4. Eat well 80% of the time. As Michael Pollen stated, "Eat food. Not too much. Mostly plants."

5. Breathe. Be mindful. Do gratitude journaling. Decrease stress.

6. Get quality sleep. Choose the right mattress and pillow. Optimize sleep hygiene.

7. Sit, drive, and work properly. Address postural ergonomics.

8. Keep your muscles in balance. Do the recommended daily exercises/stretches either from your condition in the Physical Pain Chapter or the whole body exercise program in Chapter 13. Aim to exercise three to four times a week.

9. Address trigger points early with myofascial release techniques.

10. Remove as many environmental toxins as you can afford to remove.

11. Develop a community for yourself. Surround yourself with people who make you happy. Schedule fun activities, preferably with the people who make you happy, one to two times per month.

Use the free resources available. The Internet and social media are incredible resources. There are blogs, YouTube videos, apps, and inexpensive books on Amazon dedicated to trying to make healthy living cheaper, faster, and attainable. See the Resources section for a list.

If it is financially feasible and this book does not eliminate your pain, I encourage you to find a functional medicine or integrative practitioner with a background in treating pain. If one is not available in your area, in addition to your conventional pain doctor, seek out a functional medicine practitioner. The functional medicine practitioner can identify and treat hormonal deficiencies, dysbiosis of the gut, and nutritional deficiencies, and the pain doctor can diagnose your physical pain conditions. Functional medicine is a costly investment because this care and specialty lab testing is not covered by insurance, but remember, our greatest wealth is our health.

Additionally, there are a number of interventional treatments for patients suffering from severe chronic pain—and some of these aim to heal rather than just mask symptoms, such as stem cell or platelet-rich plasma therapies (collectively known as *regenerative medicine*). Others, such as ablations, can provide much-needed long-term relief. You can seek a board-certified, fellowship-trained interventional pain physician with training in regenerative medicine for assistance.

For some of you, your pain may be so severe that you need conventional medical treatments, such as spinal cord stimulators, intrathecal pumps, or medications, to enable you to function. An interventional pain physician can help. If you use these treatments along with the lifestyle recommendations in this book, you will drastically reduce your pain as opposed to just doing the conventional treatments alone.

Have your spouse, partner, or close friends read this book so they understand why you are changing and want to change too. Make healthy living a lifestyle for your entire family.

If this book has reduced your pain (and even if it hasn't), I urge you to visit with your primary care doctor and go through your medications (prescription as well as over the counter) and see what you can eliminate from your list. Many medications have side effects, and if you do not need to be on them, it's best not to be.

As Nido Qubein said, "Your present circumstances don't determine where you can go; they merely determine where you start."

So look ahead at your pain-free future. Start small, think big, and know that one day you will look back and remember the day you broke your pain cycle.

APPENDIX: EXERCISES

To avoid injury, please first seek guidance from your physician or physical therapist prior to doing these exercises. If anything is painful, do not continue. Please do not overstretch or stretch into a painful position.

If an exercise title is starred (*Title*), a video demonstration of the exercise can be found on www.drdecaria.com/exercises/.

Here is some simple equipment you will need for these exercises:

1. A yoga mat ($13 on Amazon) or towel.

2. Yoga block (2/$10 on Amazon). Alternatively, you can use a large hardcover book or thick paperback book with a few pieces of cardboard inside. Wrap book with duct tape.

3. Bath towel.

4. 1–2 pound weights or cans of food.

5. Strap to assist with stretches ($7 on Amazon) or two neckties tied together.

EXERCISE 1: ANTERIOR CHEST STRETCH

1. Place rolled-up towel or foam roller between shoulder blades. Rest head on towel/roller. If your lower back is painful, extend the roller the length of your spine so the end of the spine and your head are both supported.

2. Spread arms out to sides, palms up, for 20–30 seconds.

3. Then bend arms at elbow, as pictured, and hold this position for 20–30 seconds. Then relax.

4. Repeat 2–3 times.

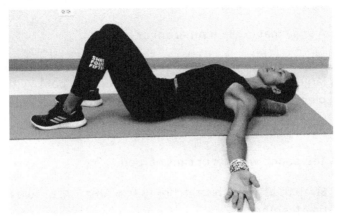

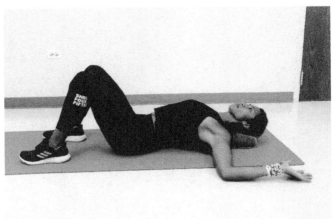

PART 2

1. Remove towel. Place one arm behind the head and the other arm out to the side. Keep legs bent and turned towards the side of the bent arm. You can place the roller between your knees to keep your pelvis steady

2. Hold this stretch for 20–30 seconds.

3. Switch arms and repeat.

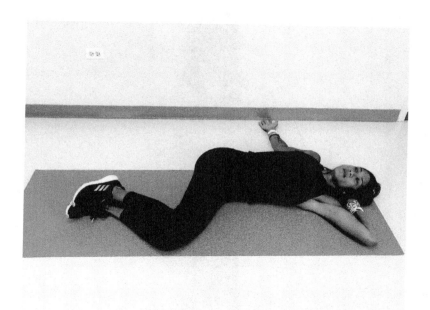

EXERCISE 2: SCAPULAR SQUEEZE

1. Bring shoulder blades back toward one another, as in the second picture.

2. Hold for 5 seconds.

3. Repeat 10–15 times.

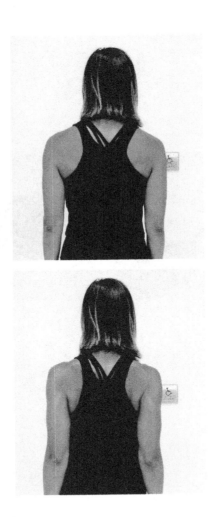

EXERCISE 3: *PRONE SCAPULAR SQUEEZE INTO LOCUST*

1. Reach your hands behind your back and interlace your fingers.

   - If unable to reach fingers, hold onto a yoga strap.

2. Squeeze shoulder blades back, allowing arms to lift.

3. Then lift your head, followed by your legs.

4. Hold and breathe slowly.

5. Work up to holding 15–20 seconds as tolerated.

6. Do twice every day.

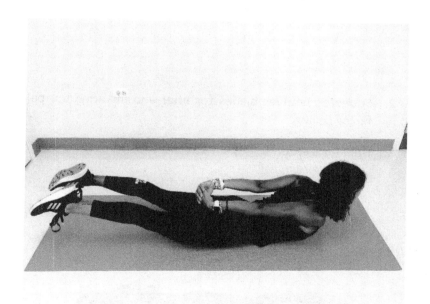

EXERCISE 4: *SCAPULAR STRENGTHENING SERIES*

1. Start with arms at side, forehead resting on a small towel roll if needed for neck comfort.

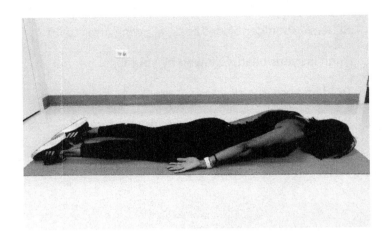

2. Squeeze shoulder blades together and lift arms up, palms facing ceiling.

3. Hold for 5 seconds. Repeat 10 times.

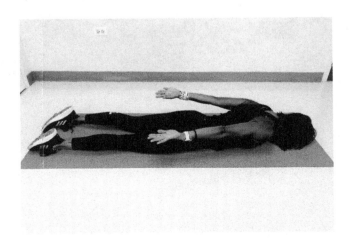

4. Then put arms out to the side, as pictured, palms facing floor. Squeeze shoulder blades back towards one another and raise your arms off the ground. Hold for 5 seconds and relax. Repeat 10 times.

5. Repeat entire set 2 more times. Do this 2–3 times per week.

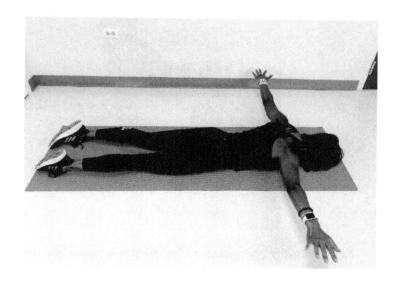

EXERCISE 5. *CAT-COW POSE*

1. Inhale, extending your spine and looking up toward the ceiling.

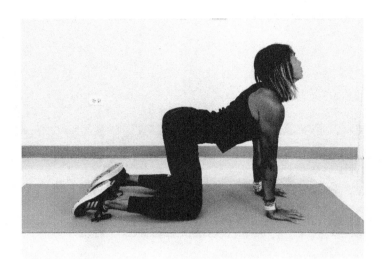

2. Exhale, flexing your spine and turning your gaze downward.

3. Repeat 10 times.

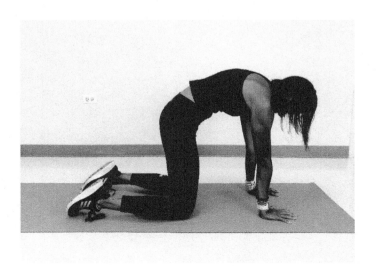

EXERCISE 6: *SHOULDER STRENGTHENING SERIES*

1. Start on your mat, on all fours.

2. Push away from mat, separating shoulder blades and activating arms. Hold for 5 seconds.

3. Then squeeze shoulder blades back together, relaxing chest toward the ground, and hold 5 seconds.

4. Repeat 10–15 times.

5. Then, while pressing through your hands and broadening your upper back, slowly shift weight slightly from side to side, pressing through the hand first on the right, then to the left while keeping the shoulder blades engaged and stable.

6. Shift back and forth 5–10 times as comfortable.

7. Repeat the entire set a second time.

8. If your wrists become uncomfortable, move onto your fists instead of your hands.

9. See video on www.drdecaria.com.

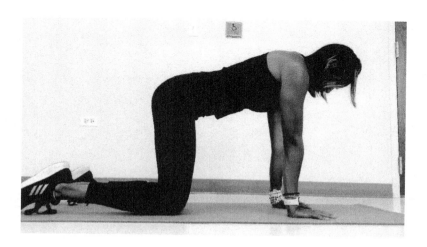

EXERCISE 7: COBRA POSE

1. Lie down on your stomach and tuck your tailbone, pressing the front of your pelvis into the ground.

2. Keeping your arms close to your side at chest level, palms on the ground, engage the gluteal and upper back muscles and lift the chest up away from the floor.

3. Hold for 10–20 seconds and then relax back to the ground.

4. Repeat 2–3 times.

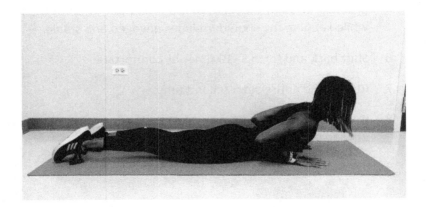

EXERCISE 8: *CHIN TUCKS*

1. Bring chin back, as if giving yourself a double chin.

2. Think about someone pulling your head straight back from the center of the back of your head, while facing forward, and/or lengthening through the crown of your head toward the ceiling.

3. You can even place fingers on your chin to make it easier.

4. Hold for 5 seconds.

5. Repeat 5–10 times.

6. Do this for postural correction at least 3–5 times throughout the day.

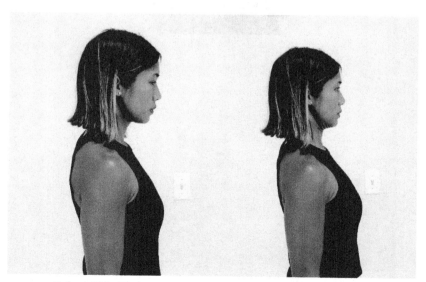

Before Chin Tuck   **After Chin Tuck**

EXERCISE 9: CARPAL TUNNEL STRETCH

1. Extend your arm in front of you with the palm up.

2. Bend wrist with the other hand, gently, until you feel a mild to moderate stretch in your forearm.

3. Hold for 20–30 seconds. Repeat 3 times.

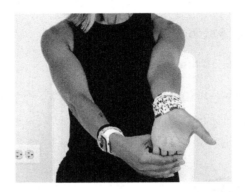

EXERCISE 10: FOREARM FLOSSING

1.   Reach your arm to the side at shoulder height, maintaining a slight bend in left elbow, palm facing ceiling.

2.   Let left ear tilt toward left shoulder. Hold for a few seconds.

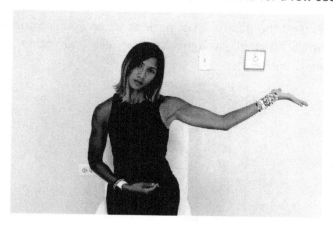

3.   Then bring arm in, bending elbow further, and tilting head to the other side.

4.   Repeat 10–15 times.

5.   This gently glides the nerve.

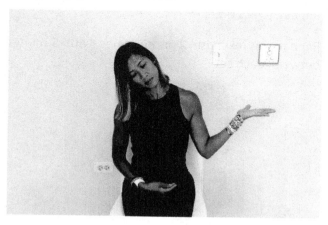

EXERCISE 11: TENNIS ELBOW ECCENTRIC EXERCISE

1. Hold a 1- to 2-pound weight in your hand.

2. Rest the painful arm on a table with your palm facing down, allowing your hand to hang off the edge.

3. Extend the painful wrist back as far as you comfortably can while lifting the weight. You can use your other hand for assistance.

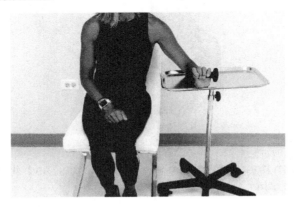

4. Slowly lower the hand with the weight in it, allowing the wrist to flex down past the edge of the table.

5. Repeat 10–15 times.

6. Repeat this exercise 2 more times with 5-minute breaks between each set.

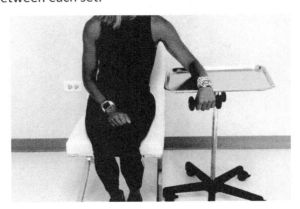

EXERCISE 12: GOLFER'S ELBOW ECCENTRIC EXERCISE

1. Hold a 1- to 2-pound weight in your hand.

2. Rest the painful arm on a table with your palm facing up, allowing your hand to hang off the edge.

3. Flex the painful wrist back as far as you comfortably can while lifting the weight. You can use your other hand for assistance.

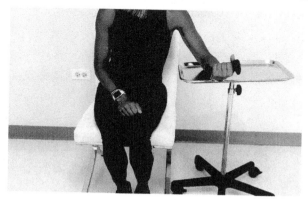

4. Slowly lower the hand with the weight in it, allowing the wrist to extend past the edge of the table.

5. Repeat 10–15 times.

6. Repeat this exercise 2 more times with 1- to 2-minute breaks between each set.

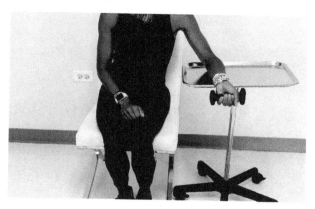

EXERCISE 13: CHILD'S POSE

1. Kneel on your hands and knees.

2. Shift your hips back until your belly rests on your legs and your forehead comes to the ground (use a small towel roll to support your head if needed), arms outstretched above you, palms on floor.

3. Rest here for 30 seconds.

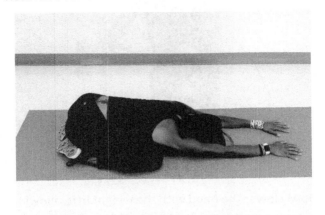

4. Then walk your arms to the right, to stretch the left side of your back, moving only your upper body. Hold for 30–60 seconds. Then repeat to the left.

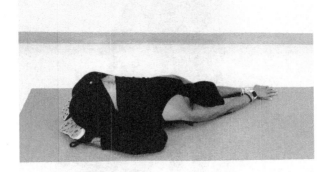

EXERCISE 14: CRESCENT MOON POSE

1. Inhale reaching your arms overhead, taking hold of your right wrist in your left hand.

2. Exhale leaning to the left and shifting your hips to the right to lengthen the right side of your body.

3. Make sure you keep steady pressure through your feet into the floor and engage your glutes to help support you in this stretch.

4. Hold for 1 minute. Then relax on an inhale back to starting position.

5. Repeat on the other side.

6. Hold for 1 minute. Repeat 2 more times for a total of 3 times a day.

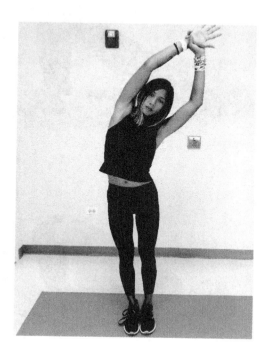

EXERCISE 15: *BRIDGE (PLUS BRIDGE WITH RESISTANCE)*

1. Start on your back, press into heels, tuck tailbone, and press up through heels to lift pelvis.

2. Hold this position 5 seconds and repeat 10–15 times to build your strength.

3. Then lower back to the ground.

4. For a higher level of difficulty, you can add a resistance band right above the knees. Once in bridge pose, you can bring thighs outwards, hold with resistance from the band for a few seconds, and then release the resistance and lower back down to the ground.

5. Repeat 10 times, 2 sets.

6. This strengthening exercise can be done 2–3 times per week.

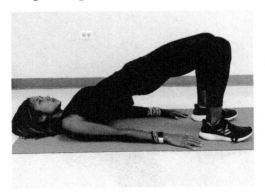

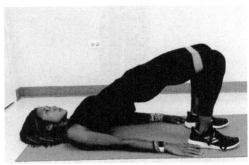

EXERCISE 16: KNEE TO CHEST TO HAMSTRING

1. This exercise is an easy way to stretch your lower back, hamstrings, and gluteal muscles.

2. Leaving one leg bent at the knee, bring the other knee toward your chest while pressing your lower back into the floor.

3. Hug the raised knee toward your chest.

4. Hold the leg in place for 20–30 seconds.

5. Then lower the leg and repeat with your other leg. You can also intensify the stretch by beginning with both legs extended on the floor instead of bending them at the knees.

6. For the second part, you will then lift your leg up to stretch your hamstring.

7. If this is too challenging, you can use a belt or yoga strap to assist with the stretch, as pictured.

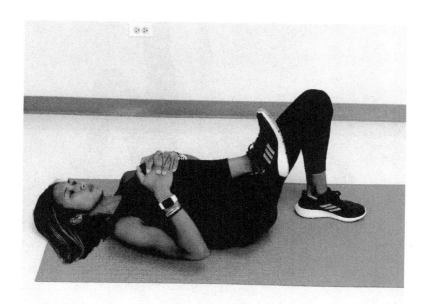

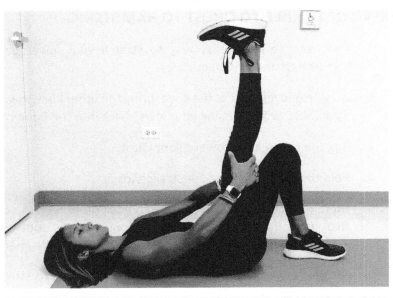

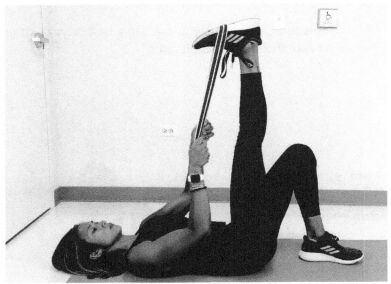

EXERCISE 17: SQUATS/KNEE TRACKING

1. Stand with your legs shoulder-width apart.

2. You can do this unassisted or with your hands lightly resting on a counter or chair in front of you.

3. Slowly bend your knees so you squat down like you are sitting in a chair.

4. Make sure your knees do not go in front of your toes and that they point the same direction as your second toe (so they don't droop in or press out).

5. Lower yourself about 6–8 inches, keeping your heels on the floor at all times.

6. At first, limit the bend of your knee to a 30-degree angle. You can slowly work up to a deeper squat. If it is causing any knee pressure or pain, do not do it.

7. Rise slowly back to a standing position.

8. Do 8–12 repetitions, 3 times per day to retrain your body in this movement.

9. You can also do 8–12 repetitions, 2–3 sets in a row 2–3x/week to build strength.

10. If your balance feels unsteady, you can stand with your hands lightly resting on a counter or chair in front of you. Place your feet shoulder-width apart.

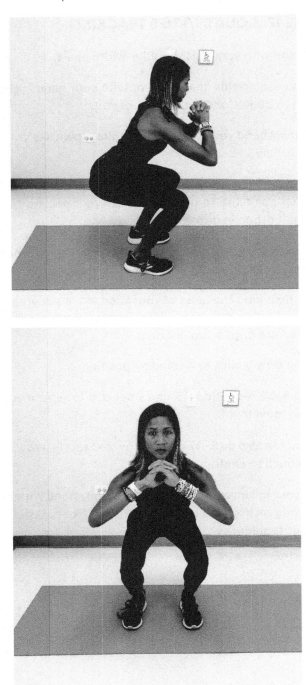

EXERCISE 18: *BENT KNEE FALL OUT*

1. Take a deep breath in.

2. As you exhale, draw your belly button back toward your spine and allow your right knee to fall gently to the side.

3. On inhale, lift the right knee back up to center.

4. Repeat 10 times on the right and 10 on the left.

5. As you get stronger, you can alternate legs—one knee out to right, followed by left as one cycle. Do 10 for each side.

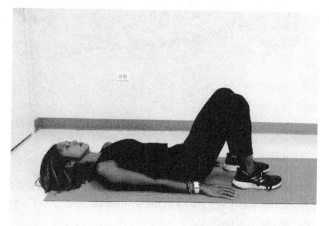

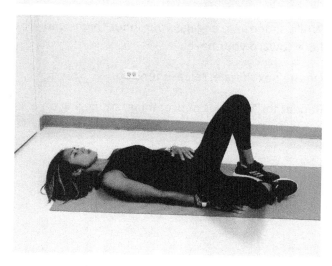

EXERCISE 19: *KNEE SQUEEZE*

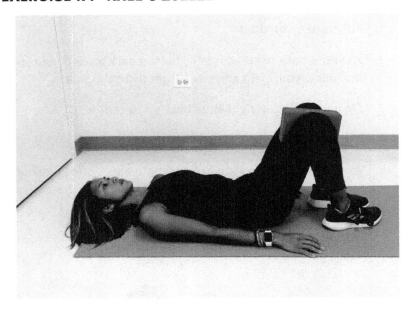

1. Inhale deeply.

2. On the exhale, draw your belly button toward your spine and simultaneously squeeze your knees together on a yoga block or rolled-up towel.

3. While squeezing, engage your inner thighs and lift the pelvic floor toward your navel.

4. On the next inhale, release tension.

5. Repeat for 10 cycles of breathing, squeezing on exhalation.

EXERCISE 20: 4-WAY HIP

1. These exercises done together will help to strengthen the muscles around your hip joint.

2. Lie on the ground. Begin by placing one foot on the ground, bent at the knee. Raise the other leg up straight. Hold for 3 seconds and lower. Repeat 10 times.

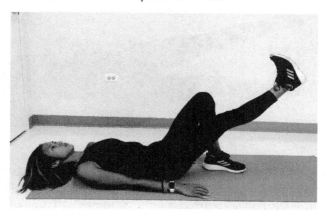

3. Then lie on your right side. Make your top leg into a 90-degree angle, as pictured, stabilizing your leg on a towel/yoga block.

4. With the other leg straight, toes pointing in front of you, lift the lower leg as far off the floor as you can. Usually a few inches is plenty. Hold for 3 seconds and lower. Repeat 10 times.

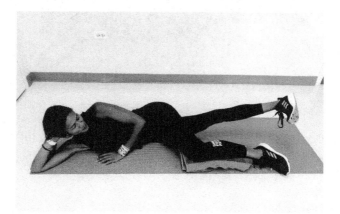

5. Lying on your right side, raise the top leg, toes pointing forward. Hold for 3 seconds and lower. Repeat 10 times.

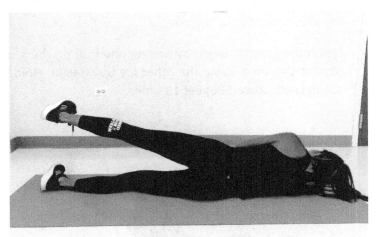

6. Then flip onto your stomach, tuck your tailbone to stabilize your pelvis, and raise your right leg up behind you. Hold for 3 seconds and lower to the ground. Repeat 10 times.

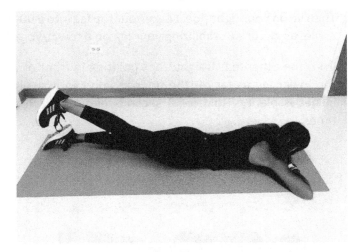

7. Do the entire set again. Repeat for the other leg (also 2 sets), 2–3 times per week.

EXERCISE 21: PSOAS STRETCH

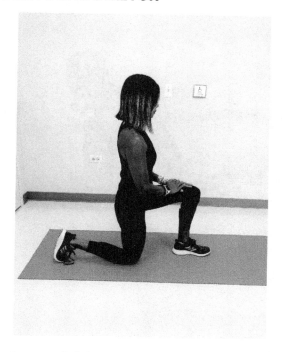

1. Keeping your left foot forward, position the left knee over the left ankle and place your right knee on the floor.

2. If this is uncomfortable, place a towel underneath your knee for added support.

3. Shift forward slightly toward the left knee, extending your right leg back as pictured. Squeeze your gluteal muscles and breathe into the hip flexor stretch for 30 seconds.

4. Switch sides.

5. If this feels like it does not elicit a stretch, you can shift farther forward, placing your hands on either side of your left foot (or on a prop such as a chair if you can't reach the floor) and shift your weight forward toward the front of your back knee. Hold 20–30 seconds.

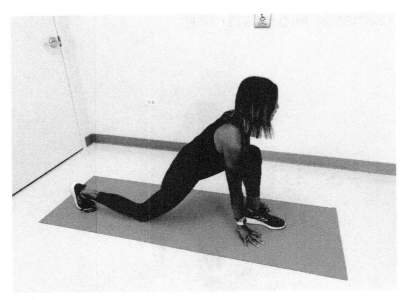

EXERCISE 22: PIRIFORMIS/HIP ABDUCTOR STRETCH

1. Lie down on your back.

2. With your left foot on the ground, knee bent, cross your right leg over the left knee to create a figure four.

3. Then place your hands behind your left thigh.

4. Using your hands, pull your right leg gently back until you feel a stretch in your piriformis. Do not overstretch, but once you feel a stretch, hold it there for 30 seconds. If this feels like too much, you can leave your left foot on the floor and gently open the right knee away from you using your right hand against your inner thigh.

5. Repeat on the other side.

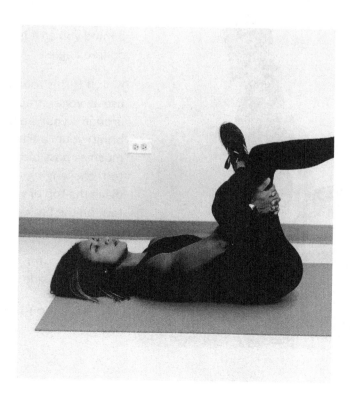

EXERCISE 23: QUAD STRETCH

1. Stand with both feet on the ground.

2. If you are unstable, you can use a wall or chair for support.

3. Bend your right knee and take hold of your right ankle, or use a strap or belt around the ankle.

4. The bent thigh should be slightly behind the other leg, or at least level with it. Feel the stretch in the front of the bent leg.

5. Bring the heel closer to the buttocks to deepen the stretch and hold for 20–30 seconds.

6. Repeat on the other side.

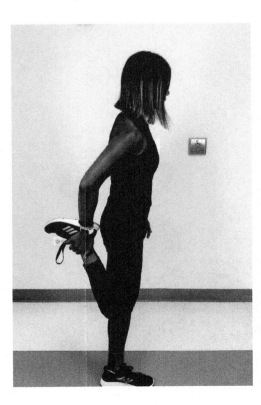

7. If this is too challenging, place the calf/leg up on a chair behind you so it is at a 90-degree angle.

8. If this is too difficult, use a yoga strap looped around your ankle to bring your ankle up as much as possible. If this is too challenging you can place the top of your right foot on the back of a chair or block.

9. Hold for 30–60 seconds per side.

10. Repeat on the other side.

VARIATION—QUAD STRETCH ON SIDE

1. Lying down on one side, bend your knee and take hold of your ankle/foot (or a strap around the ankle), bringing your heel toward your buttock.

2. Tuck your tailbone to stabilize your pelvis and spine and isolate the stretch to the front of your leg.

3. Hold for 30–60 seconds.

4. Repeat on other side

EXERCISE 24: POSTERIOR PELVIC TILT

1. Lie on your back with your knees bent. As you can see in the first photo, there is a space underneath the low back. With this exercise, we are aiming to correct that pelvic tilt and strengthen the abdominals.

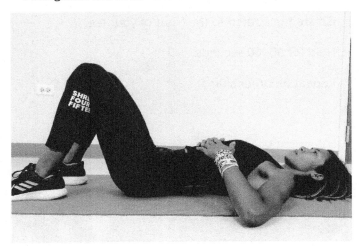

2. Flatten your back against the floor by engaging your core and tightening the abdominal muscles. You will feel as if your pelvis is bending up slightly.

3. Hold for 10 seconds. Repeat 10 times.

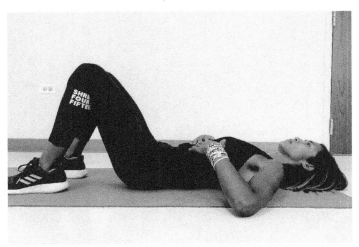

EXERCISE 25: *GLUTE ACTIVATOR*

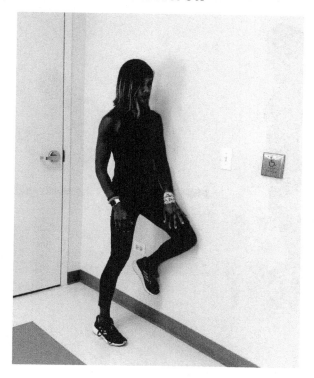

1. Start with the left side of the body against a wall.

2. Bring the left knee up as high as you can comfortably lift it. Do not lift above 90 degrees.

3. Press out against the wall and try to feel both legs activate, but particularly try to activate the hip-stabilizing muscles of the right leg.

4. If you do not feel the right leg working, you can slightly bend the right knee and sit slightly back using your right hip.

5. Start with 15 seconds and build up to a 30-second hold. Repeat on the other side.

EXERCISE 26: DEADLIFT

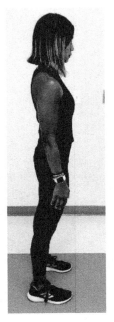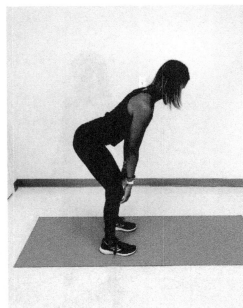

1. Stand with feet shoulder width apart, 12 inches away from a wall.

2. Hinge at hips, leaning forward keeping your back straight, reaching hips back toward the wall, keeping knees straight but soft.

3. If against a wall, you will gently tap hips to wall and then sink into your heels and use your hips to bring you back up to standing upright.

4. Repeat this 10–15 times, 2–3 sets to build strength in your hips.

5. This motion is helpful to protect your low back with movements that require you to bend forward, such as bending to the sink for personal hygiene or household chores like loading the dishwasher.

EXERCISE 27: CALF STRETCH

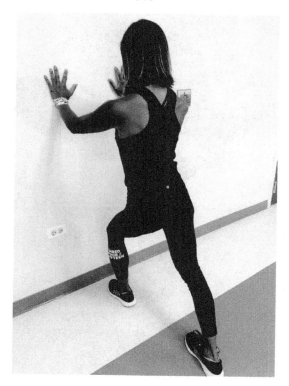

1. Stand near a wall with one foot in front of the other, front knee bent as pictured.

2. Keep your back knee straight, your heel on the ground, and lean toward the wall.

3. You should feel a stretch in the calf of your back leg.

4. Hold for 30–60 seconds.

5. Repeat on the other side.

EXERCISE 28: PERONEAL STRETCH

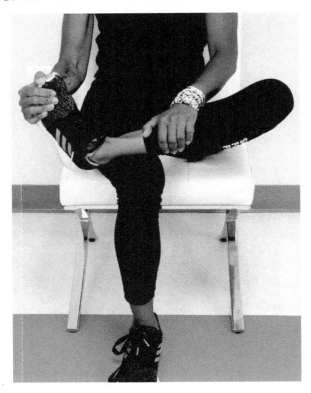

1. Sit on a chair with both feet on the ground. Bring the affected ankle up on the other knee.

2. Using your hand, lift the affected side, and turn the ankle inward as shown.

3. Hold the stretched position for 20–30 seconds and then rest.

4. Repeat 3–5 times.

EXERCISE 29: *TRIPOD FOOT POSTURE*

1. For tripod foot posture, work on creating an arch on the inside, middle part of your foot.

2. Keep the ball of the big toe on the ground and lift the inner arches, rolling toward the outside of the feet to press into the ball of your little toe while keeping the big toe on the ground.

3. You should feel three points of contact with the floor—your inner/outer front foot and middle of heel.

4. Hold 5–10 seconds, building to 30 second holds. Repeat 5 times.

5. This can be done while sitting or standing.

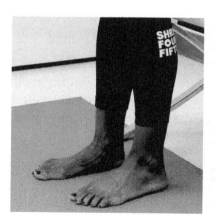 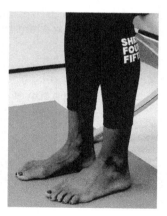

EXERCISE 30: TOE CURLS

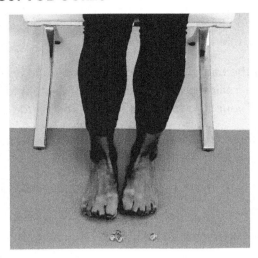

1. This is an excellent exercise to strengthen the intrinsic foot muscles.

2. You can do this in a variety of ways. You can do it with no props, with a towel that you will scrunch up with your toes, or by picking up marbles and moving them from one spot to another.

3. To do the exercise, you will keep your heel still and rest your foot on a towel.

4. Pull the towel toward you using your toes.

5. Use all five toes and try to create a dome under your arch area.

6. If you are lifting the marbles, try to create a dome or arch as you lift and move the marbles with your toes.

7. Repeat the move at least 10 times, and then repeat with the other foot. You can do this 1–2 times per day.

RESOURCES

1. **Exercise Resources**

   a. Bob & Brad Physical Therapists (www.bobandbrad.com)

   b. Yoga with Adriene (www.yogawithadriene.com)

   c. Kino Yoga, www.youtube.com/user/KinoYoga

   d. Taiflow www.taiflow.com

   e. Yoga by Candace, www.youtube.com/user/YOGABYCANDACE

2. **Websites**

   a. **Mind–Body**

      i. https://palousemindfulness.com/ (Free MBSR Course)

      ii. www.umassmed.edu/cfm/stress-reduction (Online mindfulness course)

      iii. https://www.mindbodymedicine.com/ (Dr Schechter's site)

      iv. Duke Integrative Mindfulness Based Stress Reduction Program

      v. Mindfulness-Based Chronic Pain Management (MBCPM) http://www.neuronovacentre.com

      vi. Heart Math Institute

      vii. University of Pennsylvania Positive Psychology Center

      viii. www.Research.EFTuniverse.com (evidence supporting EFT)

  b. **www.EWG.org**

  c. **Biofeedback**

      i. Biofeedback Certification International Alliance (BCIA) has searchable database of certified providers on their website: www.bcia.org; also a source for provider listing: www.aapb.org

3. **Books and Resources**

  a. **Mind-Body Syndrome Books**

      i. *Mind Body Prescription* by Dr. John Sarno

      ii. *Healing Back Pain* by Dr. Sarno

      iii. *The MindBody Workbook* by Dr. Schechter

      iv. *Unlearn Your Pain* by Howard Schubiner

      v. *The Body Keeps the Score* by Bessel van der Kolk MD

      vi. *Tapping Solution for Pain Relief* by Nick Ortner

  b. **Nutrition Books**

      i. *Your Body in Balance* by Neal Barnard, MD

      ii. *The Adrenal Reset Diet* by Alan Christianson

      iii. *8 Weeks to Optimum Health* by Andrew Weil, MD

      iv. *Your Nutrition Solution to Inflammation* by Kimberly Tessmer

      v. *Eat to Live* by Joel Fuhrman, MD

    vi.   *Food: What the Heck Should I Eat?* by Mark Hyman, MD

    vii.   *Grain Brain* by David Perlmutter, MD

    viii.   *Inflammation Spectrum* by Dr. Will Cole

    ix.   *The Microbiome Solution* by Robynne Chutkan, MD

    x.   *Clean Gut* by Alejandro Junger, MD

    xi.   *No Grain, No Pain* by Peter Osborne

    xii.   *The Gut Balance Revolution* by Gerard E. Mullin, MD

    xiii.   *The Elimination Diet* by Tom Malterre

    xiv.   https://www.pcrm.org/

    xv.   www.nutrition.gov

    xvi.   www.eatright.org

    xvii.   www.choosemyplate.gov

    xviii.   www.health.harvard.edu/glycemic

c. **Physical Pain Books**

    i.   *Back Mechanic* by Stuart McGill

    ii.   *Treat Your Own Back* by Robin A. McKenzie

d. **Resources for Supplements/Herbs/Botanicals**

    i.   https://www.nutrition.gov/topics/dietary-supplements/herbal-supplements

    ii.   https://www.nal.usda.gov/fnic/herbal-information

    iii.   National Medicines Database (https://naturalmedicines.therapeuticresearch.com/)

      iv. www.consumerlab.com

      v. https://www.nccih.nih.gov/

4. **Helpful Apps**

    a. Cronometer—Nutrition Tracker

    b. Curable health app

    c. Pocket Yoga

    d. Headspace

    e. Biozen (Android)

    f. Calm (Android, iOS)

    g. Gratitude Journal (iOS)

    h. Inner Balance (iOS)

    i. 21-Day Vegan KickStart (free)—Diet

    j. UPRIGHT GO posture analysis app

5. **Find a Practitioner**

Below you will find a list of organizations that can help guide you to find a practitioner. Please do your research to fully investigate the qualifications and training of whomever you choose.

    a. Institute of Functional Medicine: www.ifm.org/find-a-practitioner/

    b. Consortium of Academic Health Centers for Integrative Medicine www.imconsortium.org

    c. American Board of Anesthesiology to find board-certified interventional pain physicians http://www.theaba.org

    d. Certified acupuncturists: https://directory.nccaom.org/

e. Mind-body syndrome providers:
https://www.tmswiki.org/ppd/Find_a_TMS_Doctor_or_
Therapist

f. Myofascial Release Therapists

   i. John F. Barnes therapists (Barnes' therapy):
   http://mfrtherapists.com/

   ii. Dr. Ida Rolf therapists (rolfing):
   https://mms.rolf.org/members/directory/search_rol
   f_FAR.php

g. Feldenkrais

   i. www.feldenkrais.com/

ABOUT THE AUTHOR

Dr. Sheetal DeCaria is double board certified in anesthesia and pain management by the American Board of Anesthesiology. Raised in the Midwest, Dr. DeCaria attended medical school at Wayne State University in Detroit, Michigan. She then completed her anesthesia residency at the University of Chicago and interventional pain fellowship at Northwestern University. After completing her fellowship, Dr. DeCaria was on faculty at the University of Chicago, where she taught dozens of physicians in training. During this time, she pursued further education in integrative medicine, including a year-long Faculty Scholars Program at the Northwestern Osher Center for Integrative Medicine.

Since then, she has completed additional coursework through the Institute for Functional Medicine, the Academy of Integrative Pain Management, and the American Academy of Anti-Aging Medicine. In addition to serving as a medical expert for various media outlets, she has authored numerous textbook chapters and peer-reviewed publications, presented at national conferences, and serves as an expert peer reviewer for a top-tier national pain medicine journal.

In 2018, Dr. DeCaria decided to leave her academic position at the University of Chicago to open her own practice in the north suburbs of Chicago, Illinois. Her practice is split into two parts, similar to this book. Her insurance-based pain clinic is Revitalize Medical Center, and her functional medicine practice, which uses programs to optimize long-term health, is Revitalize Wellness Center. If you would like to learn more, please visit www.drdecaria.com or www.revitalizemedcenter.com.

REFERENCES

INTRODUCTION

[1] Clinical hours for anesthesia training provided by www.ASAhq.org (https://www.asahq.org/whensecondscount/wp-content/uploads/2018/01/policymaker-brochure-wsc2017_final.pdf).

[2] Henschke N, Kamper SJ, Maher CG. "The Epidemiology and Economic Consequences of Pain." *Mayo Clin Proc.* 2015; 90(1): 139–147.

[3] www.drugabuse.gov

[4] Lee M, Silverman SM, et al. "A Comprehensive Review of Opioid-induced Hyperalgesia." *Pain Physician.* 2011; 14(2): 145–161.

CHAPTER 1: THE 21ST CENTURY CHRONIC PAIN EPIDEMIC

[1] https://www.iasp-pain.org/PublicationsNews/NewsDetail.aspx?ItemNumber=10475

[2] https://www.cdc.gov/mmwr/volumes/67/wr/mm6736a2.htm

[3] "When Doctors Struggle with Suicide, Their Profession Often Fails Them." NPR.org.

CHAPTER 3: PHYSICAL PAIN SYNDROME: UNDERSTANDING YOUR DIAGNOSIS

[1] Tornbjerg SM, Nissen N, Englund M, et al. "Structural Pathology Is Not Related to Patient-reported Pain and Function in Patients Undergoing Meniscal Surgery." *Br J Sports Med*. 2017; 51(6): 525–530.

[2] Kise NJ et al. "Exercise Therapy vs. Arthroscopic Partial Meniscectomy for Degenerative Meniscal Tear in Middle-aged Patients: Randomised Controlled Trial with Two Year Follow-up." *BMJ*. 2018; 363: k4893.

[3] Paavola M, Malmivaara A, Taimela S, Kanto K, Jarvinen TL, Investigators F. "Finnish Subacromial Impingement Arthroscopy Controlled Trial (FIMPACT): A protocol for a Randomized Trial Comparing Arthroscopic Subacromial Decompression and Diagnostic Arthroscopy (placebo control), with an Exercise Therapy Control, in the Treatment of Shoulder Impingement Syndrome." *BMJ*. 2017; 7(5).

[4] Connor PM, Banks DM, Tyson AB, Coumas JS, D'Alessandro DF. "Magnetic Resonance Imaging of the Asymptomatic Shoulder of Overhead Athletes: a 5-year Follow-up Study." *Am J Sports Med*. 2003; 31(5): 724–727.

[5] Jensen MC, Brant-Zawadzki MN, Obuchowski N, Modic MT, Malkasian D, Ross JS. "Magnetic Resonance Imaging of the Lumbar Spine in People Without Back Pain." *N Engl J Med*. 1994; 331(2): 69–73.

[6] Brinjikji W, Luetmer PH, Comstock B, et al. "Systematic Literature Review of Imaging Features of Spinal Degeneration in Asymptomatic Populations." *AJNR Am J Neuroradiol*. 2015; 36(4): 811–816.

[7] Atlas SJ, Keller RB, Wu YA, Deyo RA, Singer DE. "Long-term Outcomes of Surgical and Nonsurgical Management of Lumbar

Spinal Stenosis: 8 to 10 Year Results from the Maine Lumbar Spine Study." *Spine (Phila Pa 1976)*. 2005; 30(8): 936–943.

[8] Tornbjerg SM, Nissen N, Englund M, et al. "Structural Pathology Is Not Related to Patient-reported Pain and Function in Patients Undergoing meniscal Surgery." *Br J Sports Med*. 2017; 51(6): 525–530.

[9] H.G. Fassbender and K. Wegner, "Morphologie und Pathogenese des Weichteilrheumatismus," Z. Rheumaforsch. 1973; 32: 355.

[10] Glogowski G, Wallraff J. "Ein Beitrag zur Klinik und Histologie der Muskelhärten (Myogelosen) [Clinical and histologic aspects of myogelosis]." *Z Orthop Ihre Grenzgeb*. 1951; 80(2): 237–268.

CHAPTER 4: PHYSICAL PAIN SYNDROME: CORRECT YOUR IMBALANCES

[1] Tiel RL. "Piriformis and Related Entrapment Syndromes: Myth and Fallacy." *Neurosurg Clin N Am*. 2008; 19(4): 623.

[2] Englund M, Guermazi A, Gale D, et al. "Incidental Meniscal Findings on Knee MRI in Middle-Aged and Elderly Persons." *N Engl J Med*. 2008; 359(11): 1108–1115.

[3] Agathos E, Tentolouris A, Eleftheriadou I, et al. "Effect of Alpha-lipoic Acid on Symptoms and Quality of Life in Patients with Painful Diabetic Neuropathy." *J Int Med Res*. 2018; 46(5): 1779–1790.

[4] Vallianou N, Evangelopoulos A, Koutalas P. "Alpha-lipoic Acid and Diabetic Neuropathy." *Rev Diabet Stud*. 2009; 6(4): 230–236.

CHAPTER 5: MIND-BODY PAIN SYNDROME: UNDERSTANDING THE LINK

[1] Melzack R & Wall PD. "Pain Mechanisms: A New Theory." *Science*. 1965; 19 (3699): 971–979.

[2] https://www.iasp-pain.org/PublicationsNews/NewsDetail.aspx?ItemNumber=10475

[3] Melzack R & Wall, P. (1982). "The Challenge of Pain. Harmondsworth: Penguin."

[4] Biro D. "Is there Such a Thing as Psychological Pain? And Why it Matters." *Cult Med Psychiatry*. 2010; 34(4): 658–667.

[5] Roland, M and van Tulder, M. "Should Radiologists Change the Way They Report Plain Radiography of the Spine?" *Lancet*. 1998; 352(9123): 220–230.

[6] Jarvik JG, Hollingworth W, Martin B et al. "Rapid Magnetic Resonance Imaging Vs. Radiographs for Patients with Low Back Pain: A Randomized Controlled Trial." *JAMA*. 2003; 289(21) 2810–2818.

[7] Hannan, MT et al. "Analysis of the Discordance Between Radiographic Changes and Knee Pain in Osteoarthritis of the Knee." *J Rheum*. 2000; 27: 1513–1517.

[8] Fassbender HG & Wegner K. "Morphologie und Pathogenese des Weichteilrheumatismus." *Z. Rheumaforsch*. 1973; 32: 355.

[9] Sarno, John E. "*Mind Over Back Pain: A Radically New Approach to the Diagnosis and Treatment of Back Pain*." New York: Berkeley; 1986.

[10] Sarno, J. "Etiology of Neck and Back Pain: An Autonomic Myoneuralgia?" *The Journal of Nervous and Mental Disease*. 1981; 169: 55.

[11] Splithoff CA, "Lumbosacral Junction Roentgenographic Comparison of Patients with and Without Backaches," *JAMA*. 1953; 152: 1610.

[12] Magora A. and Schwartz A., "Relation Between Low Back Pain and X-Ray Changes. 4. Lysis and Olisthesis," *Scandinavian J of Rehabilitation Medicine*. 1980; 12: 47.

[13] Schechter D, et al. "Outcomes of a Mind–body Treatment Program for Chronic Back Pain with no Distinct Structural Pathology—A Case Series of Patients Diagnosed and Treated as Tension Myositis Syndrome." *Altern Ther Health Med.* 2007; 13(5): 26–35.

[14] Schechter D, et al. "Outcomes of a Mind–body Treatment Program for Chronic Back Pain with no Distinct Structural Pathology—A Case Series of Patients Diagnosed and Treated as Tension Myositis Syndrome." *Altern Ther Health Med.* 2007; 13(5): 26–35.

[15] McEwen BS, Gianaros PJ. "Central Role of the Brain In Stress and Adaptation: Links to Socioeconomic status, Health, and Disease." *Ann N Y Acad Sci.* 2010; 1186: 190–222.

[16] Crofford LJ, Young EA, Engleberg NC et al. "Basic Circadian and Pulsatile ACTH and Cortisol Secretion in Patients with Fibromyalgia and/or Chronic Fatigue Syndrome." *Brain Behav Immun.* 2004; 18(4): 314–25.

[17] Hannibal KE, Bishop MD. "Chronic Stress, Cortisol Dysfunction, and Pain: A Psychoneuroendocrine Rationale for Stress Management in Pain Rehabilitation." *Phys Ther.* 2014; 94(12): 1816–1825.

[18] McEwen BS, Gianaros PJ. "Central Role of the Brain In Stress and Adaptation: Links to Socioeconomic status, Health, and Disease." *Ann N Y Acad Sci.* 2010; 1186: 190–222.

[19] Barsky AJ, Borus JF. "Somatization and Medicalization in the Era of Managed Care." *JAMA.* 1995; 274: 1931–4.

[20] Barsky AJ, Borus JF. "Somatization and Medicalization in the Era of Managed Care." *JAMA.* 1995; 274: 1931–4.

[21] Righter EL, Sansone RA. "Managing Somatic Preoccupation." *Am Fam Physician.* 1999; 59: 3113–20.

[22] Barsky AJ, Orav EJ, Bates DW. "Somatization Increases Medical Utilization and Costs Independent of Psychiatric and Medical Comorbidity." *Arch Gen Psychiatry*. 2005; 62: 903–10.

[23] Barsky AJ, Ettner SL, Horsky J, Bates DW. "Resource Utilization of Patients with Hypochondriacal Health Anxiety and Somatization." *Med Care*. 2001; 39: 705–15.

[24] Chaturvedi SK, Desai G, Shaligram D. "Somatoform Disorders, Somatization and Abnormal Illness Behaviour." *Int Rev Psychiatry*. 2006; 18: 75–80.

[25] Hiller W, Fichter MM, Rief W. "A Controlled Treatment Study of Somatoform Disorders Including Analysis of Healthcare Utilization and Cost-effectiveness." *J Psychosom Res*. 2003; 54: 369–80.

[26] Grassi C., Deriu F., Artusio E, Passatore M. "Modulation of the Jaw Jerk Reflex by the Sympathetic Nervous System." *Arch Ital Biol*. 1993; 131 (2-3): 213–226.

[27] Grassi C. et al. "Effect of Sympathetic Nervous System Activation on Tonic Vibration Reflex in Rabbit Jaw Closing Muscles." *J Physiol*. 1993; 469: 601–613.

[28] Grassi C., Passatore M. "Action of the Sympathetic System on Skeletal Muscle." *Ital J Neurol Sci*. 1988; 9(1): 23–28.

[29] McNulty WH, Gevirtz RN, et al. "Needle EMG Evaluation of Trigger Point Response to a Psychological Stressor." *Psychophysiology*. 1994; 31(3): 313–316.

[30] McNulty WH, Gevirtz RN, et al. "Needle EMG Evaluation of Trigger Point Response to a Psychological Stressor." *Psychophysiology*. 1994; 31(3): 313–316.

[31] Banks S, Jacobs D, Gevirtz R, Hubbard D. "Effects of Autogenic Relaxation Training on EMG Activity in Active Myofascial Trigger Points." *J of Musculosketal Pain*. 1998; 64 (4): 23–32.

[32] Armm J, Gevertz R et al. "The Relationship Between Personality Characteristic and Local Muscle Tenderness Development in First Year Psychology Graduate Students: A Prospective Study." *Applied Psychophysiology and Biofeedback*. 1999; 24(2): 125.

[33] Sapolsky R. et al. "The Neuroendocrinology of Stress and Aging: The Glucocorticoid Cascade Hypothesis." *Endocr Rev*. 1986; 7: 284–301.

[34] Biro D. "Is There Such a Thing as Psychological Pain? And Why it Matters." *Cult Med Psychiatry*. 2010; 34(4): 658–667.

[35] Eisenberger NL, Lieberman MD, Williams KD. "Does Rejection Hurt? An fMRI Study of Social Exclusion." *Science*. 2003; 302: 290–292.

[36] Gündel H, O'Connor MF, Littrell L, Fort C, Lane RD. "Functional Neuroanatomy of Grief: An fMRI Study." *Am J Psychiatry*. 2003; 160(11): 1946–1953.

[37] Shimo K, Ueno T, Younger J, et al. "Visualization of Painful Experiences Believed to Trigger the Activation of Affective and Emotional Brain Regions in Subjects with Low Back Pain." *PLoS One*. 2011; 6(11).

[38] Burns JW, Holly A, Quartana P, Wolff B, Gray E, Bruehl S. "Trait Anger Management Style Moderates Effects of Actual ("State") Anger Regulation on Symptom-specific Reactivity and Recovery Among Chronic Low Back Pain Patients." *Psychosom Med*. 2008; 70(8): 898–905.

[39] Kross E, Berman MG, Mischel W, Smith EE, Wager TD. "Social Rejection Shares Somatosensory Representations with Physical Pain." *Proc Natl Acad Sci USA*. 2011; 108(15): 6270–6275.

[40] Serrano-Ibanez ER et al. "Behavioral Inhibition and Activation Systems, and Emotional Regulation in Individuals with Chronic Musculoskeletal Pain." *Front Psychiatry*. 2018; 10(9): 394.

[41] McEwen BS. "Physiology and Neurobiology of Stress and Adaptation: Central Role of the Brain." *Physiol Rev*. 2007; 87: 873–904.

[42] Arborelius L, and Eklund, MB. "Both Long and Brief Maternal Separation Produces Persistent Changes in Tissue Levels of Brain Monoamines in Middle-aged Female Rats." *Neuroscience*. 2007; 145, 738–750.

[43] Anda RF, Felitti VJ, Bremner JD, et al. "The Enduring Effects of Abuse and Related Adverse Experiences in Childhood. A Convergence of Evidence from Neurobiology and Epidemiology." *Eur Arch Psychiatry Clin Neurosci*. 2006; 256(3): 174–186.

[44] Chaloner A, Greenwood-Van Meerveld B. "Early Life Adversity as a Risk Factor for Visceral Pain in Later Life: Importance of Sex Differences." *Front Neurosci*. 2013; 7: 13.

[45] You DS, Meagher MW. "Childhood Adversity and Pain Sensitization." *Psychosomatic medicine*. 2016; 78: 1084–93.

[46] Gordon JL, Johnson J, Nau S, Mechlin B, Girdler SS. "The Role of Chronic Psychosocial Stress in Explaining Racial Differences in Stress Reactivity and Pain Sensitivity." *Psychosomatic medicine*. 2017; 79: 201–12.

[47] Tsur N, Defrin R, Ginzburg K. "Posttraumatic Stress Disorder, Orientation to Pain, and Pain Perception in Ex-Prisoners of War Who Underwent Torture." *Psychosomatic medicine*. 2017; 79: 655–63.

[48] Fishbain DA, et al. "Chronic Pain Types Differ in their Reported Prevalence of PTSD and there is Consistent Evidence that Chronic Pain is Associated with PTSD: An Evidence-Based Structured Systematic Review." 2017; 18(4): 711–735.

[49] Asmundson GJ, Coons MJ, Taylor S, Katz J. "PTSD and the Experience of Pain: Research and Clinical Implications of Shared Vulnerability and Mutual Maintenance Models." *Canadian J Psychiatry*. 2002; 47: 930–7.

[50] Scioli-Salter ER, Forman DE, Otis JD, et al. "The Shared Neuroanatomy and Neurobiology of Comorbid Chronic Pain and PTSD: Therapeutic Implications." *Clin J Pain.* 2015; 31: 363–74.

[51] Duric V, Clayton S, Leong ML, Yuan LL. "Comorbidity Factors and Brain Mechanisms Linking Chronic Stress and Systemic Illness." *Neural Plast.* 2016; 5460732.

[52] Duric V, Clayton S, Leong ML, Yuan LL. "Comorbidity Factors and Brain Mechanisms Linking Chronic Stress and Systemic Illness." *Neural Plast.* 2016; 5460732.

[53] Quartana PJ, Burns JW, Lofland KR. "Attentional Strategy Moderates Effects of Pain Catastrophizing on Symptom-specific Physiological Responses in Chronic Low Back Pain Patients." *J Behav Med.* 2007; 30(3): 221–231.

[54] Obelieniene D, Schrader H, Bovim G, Miseviciene I, Sand T. "Pain After Whiplash: A Prospective Controlled Inception Cohort Study." *J Neurol Neurosurg Psychiatry.* 1999; 66(3): 279–283.

[55] Ferrari R, Schrader H. "The Late Whiplash Syndrome: A Biopsychosocial Approach." *J Neurol Neurosurg Psychiatry.* 2001; 70(6): 722–726.

[56] Reynolds DL, Chambers LW, Badley EM, et al. "Physical Disability Among Canadians Reporting Musculoskeletal Diseases." *J Rheumatol.* 1992; 19(7): 1020–1030.

[57] White KP et al. "The London Fibromyalgia Epidemiology Study: The Prevalence of Fibromyalgia in London, Ontario." *J Rheumatol.* 1999. 26(7): 1570–1576.

[58] Asmundson GJ, Katz J. "Understanding the Co-occurrence of Anxiety Disorders and Chronic Pain: State-of-the-art." *Depress Anxiety.* 2009; 26: 888–901.

CHAPTER 6: MIND-BODY PAIN SYNDROME: RETRAIN YOUR PAIN BRAIN

[1] López-Solà C, Bui M, Hopper JL, et al. "Predictors and Consequences of Health Anxiety Symptoms: A Novel Twin Modeling Study". *Acta Psychiatr Scand*. 2018; 137(3): 241–251.

[2] Lewandowski W, Good M, Draucker CB. "Changes in the Meaning of Pain with the Use of Guided Imagery." *Pain management nursing: Official journal of the American Society of Pain Management Nurses*. 2005; 6: 58–67.

[3] López-Solà C, Bui M, Hopper JL, et al. "Predictors and Consequences of Health Anxiety Symptoms: A Novel Twin Modeling Study". *Acta Psychiatr Scand*. 2018; 137(3): 241–251.

[4] Lewandowski W, Good M, Draucker CB. "Changes in the Meaning of Pain with the Use of Guided Imagery." *Pain management nursing: Official journal of the American Society of Pain Management Nurses*. 2005; 6: 58–67.

[5] Burton C. "Beyond Somatisation: A Review of the Understanding and Treatment of Medically Unexplained Physical Symptoms (MUPS)." *Br J Gen Pract*. 2003; 53: 231–9.

[6] Barsky AJ, Ahern DK. "Cognitive Behavior Therapy for Hypochondriasis: A Randomized Controlled Trial." *JAMA*. 2004; 291: 1464–70.

[7] Allen LA, Woolfolk RL, Escobar JI, Gara MA, Hamer RM. "Cognitive-behavioral Therapy for Somatization Disorder: A Randomized Controlled Trial." *Arch Intern Med*. 2006; 166: 1512–8.

[8] Van der Feltz-Cornelis CM, van Oppen P, Ader HJ, van Dyck R. "Randomised Controlled Trial of a Collaborative Care Model with Psychiatric Consultation for Persistent Medically Unexplained Symptoms in General Practice." *Psychother Psychosom*. 2006; 75: 282–9.

[9] Dutcher JM et al. "Neural Mechanisms of Self-affirmation's Stress Buffering Effects." Social Cognitive and Affective Neuroscience. 2020.

[10] Ma X. et al. "The Effect of Diaphragmatic Breathing on Attention, Negative Affect, and Stress in Healthy Adults." Front Psychol. 2017; 8: 874.

[11] Mastorakos G, Pavlatou M, Diamanti-Kandarakis E, Chrousos GP. "Exercise and the Stress System." *Hormones (Athens)*. 2005; 4(2): 73–89.

[12] Fishman L., Saltonstall E. (2008) Yoga in Pain Management. In: Audette J.F., Bailey A. (eds) Integrative Pain Medicine: The Science and Practice of Complementary and Alternative Medicine in Pain Management. Humana Press.

[13] Solloway MR, Taylor SL, Shekelle PG, et al. "An Evidence Map of the Effect of Tai Chi on Health Outcomes." *Syst Rev.* 2016; 5(1):126.

[14] Kong LJ et al. "Tai Chi for Chronic Pain Conditions: A Systematic Review and Meta-analysis of Randomized Controlled Trials." *Sci Rep.* 2016; 6: 25325.

[15] Gatchel RJ, Robinson RC, Pulliam C., Maddrey AM. "Biofeedback with Pain Patients: Evidence for its Effectiveness." *Seminars in Pain Medicine.* 2003; 1(2): 55–66.

[16] Toby RO, Newton-John SH, Spence DS. "Cognitive-behavioral Therapy Vs. EMG Biofeedback in the Treatment of Chronic Low Back Pain." *Behaviour Research and Therapy.* 1995; 33(6): 691–697.

[17] Rokicki LA, Holroyd KA, France CR, Lipchick GL, et al. "Change Mechanisms Associated with Combined Relaxation/EMG Biofeedback Training for Chronic Tension Headache." *Applied Psychophysiology and Biofeedback.* 1997; 22(1): 21–41.

[18] Crider A, Glaros AG, Gebirtz R. "Efficacy of Biofeedback-based Treatments for Temporomandibular Disorders." *Applied Psychophysiology and Biofeedback.* 2005; 30(4): 333–345.

[19] Gatchel RJ, Robinson RC, Pulliam C., Maddrey AM. "Biofeedback with Pain Patients: Evidence for its Effectiveness." *Seminars in Pain Medicine.* 2003; 1(2): 55–66.

[20] Sime a. "Case Study of Trigeminal Neuralgia Using Neurofeedback and Peripheral Biofeedback." *Journal of Neurotherapy.* 2004, 8(1): 59–71.

[21] Jensen MP, Grierson C, Tracy-Smith V, et al. "Neurofeedback Treatment for Pain Associated with Complex Regional Pain Syndrome Type 1." *Journal of Neurotherapy.* 2007; 11(1): 45–53.

[22] Kayiran s, Dursun E, Dursun N et al. "Neurofeedback Intervention in Fibromyalgia Syndrome; A Randomized, Controlled Clinical Trial." *Applied Psychophysiology and Biofeedback.* 2010; 35(4): 293–302.

CHAPTER 7: CENTRAL PAIN SYNDROME: HEALING BRAIN AND BODY INFLAMMATION

[1] Littlejohn G. "Neurogenic Neuroinflammation in Fibromyalgia and Complex Regional Pain Syndrome." *Nat Rev Rheumatol.* 2015; 11(11): 639–48.

[2] Littlejohn G. "Neurogenic Neuroinflammation in Fibromyalgia and Complex Regional Pain Syndrome." *Nat Rev Rheumatol.* 2015; 11(11): 639–48.

[3] Robinson M, Craggs J. et al. "Gray Matter Volumes of Pain Related Brain Areas are Decreased in Fibromyalgia Syndrome." *J Pain.* 2011; 12(4): 436–443.

[4] Cordero, MD, De Miguel, M, Moreno Fernández, AM, *et al.* "Mitochondrial Dysfunction and Mitophagy Activation in Blood

Mononuclea Cells of Fibromyalgia Patients: Implications in the Pathogenesis of the Disease." *Arthritis Res Ther.* 2010; 12, R17.

[5] Tan EC et al. "Mitochondrial Dysfunction in Muscle Tissue of CRPS Type I Patients." *Eur J Pain.* 2011; 15(7): 708–715.

[6] Gerdle et al. "Chronic Widespread Pain: Increased Glutamate and Lactate Concentrations in the Trapezius Muscle and Plasma." *Clin J Pain.* 2014; 30(5): 409–20.

[7] Buskila D, Atzeni F, Sarzi-Puttini P. "Etiology of Fibromyalgia:The Possible Role of Infection and Vaccination." *Autoimmun Rev.* 2008; 8(1): 41–43.

[8] Frissora CL, Koch KL. "Symptom Overlap and Comorbidity of Irritable bowel Syndrome with Other Conditions." *Curr Gastroenterol Rep.* 2005; 7(4): 264–71.

[9] Chia JK, Chia AY. "Chronic Fatigue Syndrome is Associated with Chronic Enterovirus Infection of the Stomach." *J Clin Pathol.* 2008; 61(1): 43–48.

[10] Chia JK, Chia AY. "Chronic Fatigue Syndrome is Associated with Chronic Enterovirus Infection of the Stomach." *J Clin Pathol.* 2008; 61(1): 43–48.

[11] Goebel A. "Immune Activation and Autoimmunity in Chronic Pain Conditions and Response to Immunoglobulin G." *Clin Exp Immunol.* 2014; 178: 39–41.

[12] Chenard CA, Rubenstein LM, Snetselaar LG, Wahls TL. "Nutrient Composition Comparison between a Modified Paleolithic Diet for Multiple Sclerosis and the Recommended Healthy U.S.-Style Eating Pattern." *Nutrients.* 2019; 11(3): 537.

[13] Macia L. et al. "Microbial Influences on Epithelial Integrity and Immune Function as a Basis for Inflammatory Diseases." *Immunological Reviews.* 2012; 245: 164–76.

[14] Galland L. "The gut Microbiome and the Brain." *J Med Food.* 2014; 17(12): 1261–72.

[15] Milling S. et al. "Physiological Role of Gut Microbiota." *Current Opinion in Rheumatology.* 2016; 28: 161–67.

[16] Chedid V, Dhalla S, Clarke JO, et al. "Herbal Therapy is Equivalent to Rifaximin for the Treatment of Small Intestinal Bacterial Overgrowth." *Glob Adv Health Med.* 2014; 3(3): 16–24.

[17] Milling S. et al. "Physiological Role of Gut Microbiota." *Current Opinion in Rheumatology.* 2016; 28: 161–67.

[18] Srinivasan V. et al. "Potential Use of Melatonergic Drugs in Analgesia: Mechanisms of Action." *Brain Res Bull.* 2010; 81: 362–371.

[19] Chen WW, Zhang X, Huang WJ. "Pain Control by Melatonin: Physiological and Pharmacological Effects." *Exp Ther Med.* 2016; 12(4): 1963–1968.

[20] Lattanzio SM. "Fibromyalgia Syndrome: A Metabolic Approach Grounded in Biochemistry for the Remission of Symptoms." *Front Med (Lausanne).* 2017; 4: 198.

[21] Rosenkranz et al. "A Comparison of Mindfulness-based Stress Reduction and an Active Control in Modulation of Neurogenic inflammation. *Brain Behavior, and Immunity.* 2013; 27(1): 174–184.

[22] Leung MK et al. "Increased Grey Matter Volume in the Right Angular and Posterior Parahippocampal gyri in Loving-Kindness Meditators." *Soc Cogn Affect Neurosci.* 2013; 8(1) 34–39.

[23] Tennant F, Hermann L. "Using Biological Markers to Identify the Legitimate Chronic Pain Patient." *Amer Clin Lab.* 2002; 8–17.

[24] Aloisi AM, Bonifazi M. "Sex Hormones, Central Nervous System and Pain." *Hormones and Behavior.* 2006; 50 (1): 1–7.

[25] Vuong C, Van Urim SHM et al. "The Effects of Opioids and Opioid Analogs in Animal and Human Endocrine Systems." *Endocrin Rev.* 2010; 31: 98–132.

[26] Kerstin Klein and Steffen Gay, "Epigenetics in Rheumatoid Arthritis," *Current Opinion in Rheumatology*. 2015; 27: 76–82.

[27] Maurer AJ, Lissounov A, Knezevic I, Candido KD, Knezevic NN. "Pain and Sex Hormones: A Review of Current Understanding." *Pain Manag*. 2016; 6(3): 285–296.

[28] Maurer AJ, Lissounov A, Knezevic I, Candido KD, Knezevic NN. "Pain and Sex Hormones: A Review of Current Understanding." *Pain Manag*. 2016; 6(3): 285–296.

[29] Rosen S, Ham B, Mogil JS. "Sex Differences in Neuroimmunity and Pain." *J Neurosci Res*. 2017; 95(1-2): 500–508.

[30] Sutherland AM, Clarke HA, Katz J, Katznelson R. "Hyperbaric Oxygen Therapy: A New Treatment for Chronic Pain?" *Pain Pract*. 2016 ;16(5): 620–628.

[31] Barilaro G, Francesco Masala I, Parracchini R, et al. "The Role of Hyperbaric Oxygen Therapy in Orthopedics and Rheumatological Diseases." *Isr Med Assoc J*. 2017; 19(7): 429–434.

[32] Efrati S, Golan H, Bechor Y, et al. "Hyperbaric Oxygen Therapy can Diminish Fibromyalgia Syndrome—Prospective Clinical Trial." *PLoS One*. 2015; 10(5): e0127012.

[33] Gomes da Silva S, Simoes S et al. "Exercise Induced Hippocampal Anti-inflammatory Response in Aged Rats." *J Neuroinflammation*. 2013; 10:61.

[34] Busch AJ, Webber SC, Brachaniec M, et al. "Exercise Therapy for Fibromyalgia." *Curr Pain Headache Rep*. 2011; 15(5): 358–367.

[35] Lener MS, Kadriu B, Zarate CA Jr. "Ketamine and Beyond: Investigations into the Potential of Glutamatergic Agents to Treat Depression." *Drugs*. 2017; 77(4): 381–401.

[36] Patil S, Anitescu M. "Efficacy of Outpatient Ketamine Infusions in Refractory Chronic Pain Syndromes: A 5-Year Retrospective Analysis." *Pain Med*. 2012; 13(2): 263–269.

[37] Zhu W, Ding Z, Zhang Y, Shi J, Hashimoto K, Lu L. "Risks Associated with Misuse of Ketamine as a Rapid-Acting Antidepressant." *Neurosci Bull*. 2016; 32(6): 557–564.

[38] Nutile-McMenemy N et al. "Minocycline Decreases in Vitro Microglial Motility, Beta 1 Integrin, and Kv1.3 Channel Expression." *J Neurochem*. 2007; 103(5): 2035–2046.

[39] Wang Q et al. "Naloxone Inhibits Immune Cell Function by Suppressing Superoxide Production Through a Direct Interaction with gp91phox Subunit of NADPH Oxidase." *J Neuroinflammation*. 2012; 9: 32.

[40] Patten DK, Schultz BG, Berlau DJ. "The Safety and Efficacy of Low-Dose Naltrexone in the Management of Chronic Pain and Inflammation in Multiple Sclerosis, Fibromyalgia, Crohn's Disease, and Other Chronic Pain Disorders." *Pharmacotherapy*. 2018; 38(3): 382–389.

CHAPTER 8: INTEGRATIVE HEALING OF MIND-BODY-SPIRIT

[1] American Pain Foundation (2008) Overview of American Pain Surveys: 2005–2006, Journal of Pain & Palliative Care Pharmacotherapy, 22:1, 33–38.

[2] Descalzi G, Ikegami D, Ushijima T, Nestler EJ, Zachariou V, Narita M. "Epigenetic Mechanisms of Chronic Pain." *Trends Neurosci*. 2015; 38(4): 237–246.

[3] Liang L, Lutz BM, Bekker A, Tao YX. "Epigenetic Regulation of Chronic Pain." *Epigenomics*. 2015; 7(2): 235–245.

[4] Lessans S, Dorsey SG. The role for Epigenetic Modifications in Pain and Analgesia Response." *Nurs Res Pract*. 2013; 961493.

[5] Buchheit T, Van de Ven T, Shaw A. "Epigenetics and the Transition from Acute to Chronic Pain." *Pain Med*. 2012; 13(11): 1474–1490.

CHAPTER 9. ELIMINATE THE INFLAMMATORY SOURCE

[1] Losurdo G, Principi M, Iannone A, et al. "Extra-intestinal Manifestations of Non-celiac Gluten Sensitivity: An Expanding Paradigm." *World J Gastroenterol*. 2018; 24(14): 1521–1530.

[2] Bordoni A, Danesi F, Dardevet D, et al. "Dairy Products and Inflammation: A Review of the Clinical Evidence." *Crit Rev Food Sci Nutr*. 2017; 57(12): 2497–2525.

[3] Grant EC. "Food Allergy and Migraine." *Lancet*. 1979; 2(8138): 358–359.

CHAPTER 10: FOOD AS THE FOUNDATION OF WELLNESS

[1] Christ A, Lauterbach M, Latz E. "Western Diet and the Immune System: An Inflammatory Connection." *Immunity*. 2019; 51(5): 794–811.

[2] Monti D, Ostan R, Borelli V, Castellani G, Franceschi C. "Inflammaging and Human Longevity in the Genomics Era." *Mech Ageing Dev*. 2017; 165: 129–138.

[3] Wang Z, Nakayama T. "Inflammation, a Link Between Obesity and Cardiovascular Disease." *Mediators Inflamm*. 2010; 2010: 535918.

[4] Stavropoulou E, Bezirtzoglou E. "Human Microbiota in Aging and Infection: A Review." *Crit Rev Food Sci Nutr*. 2019; 59(4): 537–545.

[5] Totsch SK, Quinn TL, Strath LJ, et al. "The Impact of the Standard American Diet in Rats: Effects on Behavior, Physiology and Recovery from Inflammatory Injury." *Scand J Pain*. 2017; 17: 316–324.

[6] Rinninella E, Raoul P, Cintoni M, et al." What is the Healthy Gut Microbiota Composition? A Changing Ecosystem across Age, Environment, Diet, and Diseases." *Microorganisms*. 2019; 7(1): 14.

[7] de Cabo R, Mattson MP. "Effects of Intermittent Fasting on Health, Aging, and Disease." *N Engl J Med*. 2020; 16; 382(3).

CHAPTER 11: FIGHTING PAIN THE NATURAL WAY: SUPPLEMENTS THAT WORK

[1] Yu et al. "Chronic Supplementation of Curcumin Enhances the Efficiency of Antidepressants in Major Depressive Disorder: A Randomized, Double Blind, Placebo Controlled Pilot Study." *J Clin Psychopharm*. 2015; 35(4): 406–410.

[2] Yu et al. "Chronic Supplementation of Curcumin Enhances the Efficiency of Antidepressants in Major Depressive Disorder: A Randomized, Double Blind, Placebo Controlled Pilot Study." *J Clin Psychopharm*. 2015; 35(4): 406–410.

[3] Bright JJ. Curcumin and Autoimmune Disease." *Adv Exp Med Biol*. 2007; 595: 425–51.

[4] Schoenen J et al. "Effectiveness of High-dose Riboflavin in Migraine Prophylaxis. A Randomized Controlled Trial." Neurology. 1998; 50: 466–70.

[5] Liem A, Reynierse-Buitenwerf GH, Zwinderman AH, et al. "Secondary Prevention with Folic Acid: Effects on Clinical Outcomes." *J Am Coll Cardiol*. 2003; 41: 2105–13.

[6] Fonseca VA et al. "Metanx in Type 2 Diabetes with Peripheral Neuropathy: A Randomized Trial." *Am J Med*. 2013; 126(2): 141–9.

[7] Bennink, H. J. and Schreurs, W. H. "Improvement of Oral Glucose Tolerance in Gestational Diabetes by Pyridoxine." *Br Med J*. 1975; 3(5974): 13–15.

[8] Natural Medicines Database

[9] Natural Medicines Database

[10] Natural Medicines Database

[11] Rohini Terry, PhD, Paul Posadzki, PhD, Leala K. Watson, BSc (Hons), Edzard Ernst, MD, PhD. "The Use of Ginger (*Zingiber officinale*) for the Treatment of Pain: A Systematic Review of Clinical Trials." *Pain Medicine*, 2011; 1808–1818.

[12] Frondoza et al. "Ginger Extract Reduced Inflammation in Synovial Cell Cultures." *In Vitro Cell Dev.* 2004; 40(3-4): 95–101.

[13] Grzanna R. et al. "Ginger Inhibits COX and LOX Pathways." *J Med Food.* 2005; 8: 125–132.

[14] Natural Medicines Database

[15] Cleland LG, et al. "The Role of Fish Oils in the Treatment of RA." *Drugs.* 2003; 63: 845–53.

[16] Fairfield, K." Vitamins for Chronic Disease Prevention in Adults, Scientific Review." *JAMA.* 2002; 287: 3116–3126.

[17] Park C, Brietzke E, Rosenblat JD, et al. "Probiotics for the Treatment of Depressive Symptoms: An Anti-inflammatory Mechanism?" *Brain Behav Immun.* 2018; 73: 115–124.

[18] Roman P, Abalo R, Marco EM, Cardona D. "Probiotics in Digestive, Emotional, and Pain-related Disorders." *Behav Pharmacol.* 2018; 29: 103–119.

[19] Lee SH, Kwon JY, Jhun J, et al." Lactobacillus Acidophilus Ameliorates pain and Cartilage Degradation in Experimental Osteoarthritis." *Immunol Lett.* 2018; 203: 6–14.

[20] Natural Medicines Database

[21] Peikert A, Wilimzig C, Kohne-Volland R. "Prophylaxis of Migraine with Oral Magnesium: Results from a Prospective, Multi-center, Placebo-controlled and Double-blind Randomized Study." *Cephalalgia.* 1996; 16: 257–63.

[22] Russell IJ, Michalek JE, Flechas JD, Abraham GE. "Treatment of Fibromyalgia Syndrome with Super Malic: A Randomized, Double-

Blind, Placebo-controlled, Crossover Pilot Study." *J Rheumatol.* 1995; 22: 953–8.

[23] Ziegler D. "ALADIN Study." *Diabetologia.* 1995; 38: 1425–33.

[24] Veresiu IA. "Treatment of Diabetic Polyneuropathy with Alpha-lipoic Acid is Evidence Based." *Rom J Intern Med.* 2004; 42: 293–99.

[25] Natural Medicines Database

[26] Natural Medicines Database

[27] Helde-Frankling M, Björkhem-Bergman L. "Vitamin D in Pain Management." *Int J Mol Sci.* 2017; 18(10): 2170.

[28] Ames B, N. "A Role for Supplements in Optimizing Health: The Metabolic Tuneup." *Arch Biochem Biophys.* 2004; 423 (1): 227–234.

[29] Danilov A, Kurganova J. "Melatonin in Chronic Pain Syndromes. *Pain Ther.*" 2016; 5(1): 1–17.

[30] Kaur T, Shyu BC. "Melatonin: A New-Generation Therapy for Reducing Chronic Pain and Improving Sleep Disorder-Related Pain." *Adv Exp Med Biol.* 2018; 1099: 229–251.

[31] Natural Medicines Database

[32] Saini R. "Coenzyme Q10: The Essential Nutrient." *J Pharm Bioallied Sci.* 2011; 3(3): 466–467.

[33] Natural Medicines Database

[34] Natural Medicines Database

[35] Tardiolo G, Bramanti P, Mazzon E. "Overview on the Effects of *N*-Acetylcysteine in Neurodegenerative Diseases." *Molecules.* 2018; 23(12): 3305.

[36] Chiechio S et al. "Acetyl L Carnitine in Neuropathic Pain." *CNS Drugs.* 2007; 21: 31–26.

[37] Rossini M et al. "Double-blind, Multicenter Trial Comparing Acetyl L Carnitine with Placebo in Treatment Fibromyalgia Patients." *Clin Exp Rheum.* 2007; 25: 182–188.

[38] Zhu X, Sang L, Wu D, Rong J, Jiang L. "Effectiveness and Safety of Glucosamine and Chondroitin for the Treatment of Osteoarthritis: A Meta-analysis of Randomized Controlled Trials." *J Orthop Surg Res.* 2018; 13(1): 170.

[39] Simental-Mendía M, Sánchez-García A, Vilchez-Cavazos F, Acosta-Olivo CA, Peña-Martínez VM, Simental-Mendía LE. "Effect of Glucosamine and Chondroitin Sulfate in Symptomatic Knee Osteoarthritis: A Systematic Review and Meta-Analysis of Randomized Placebo-controlled Trials." *Rheumatol Int.* 2018; 38(8): 1413–1428.

CHAPTER 13: WHOLE BODY STRENGTH AND WELLNESS

[1] Parsons, T.J et al. "Physical Activity, Sedentary Behavior, and Inflammatory and Hemostatic Markers in Men." *Med. Sci. Sports Exerc.* 2017; 49, 459–465.

CHAPTER 14: MINDFULNESS MAGIC

[1] Gorczyca R, Filip R, Walczak E. "Psychological Aspects of Pain." *Ann Agric Environ Med.* 2013; 20(1): 23–27.

[2] May A. "Chronic Pain May change the Structure of the Brain." *Pain.* 2008; 137: 7–15.

[3] Kuchinad A, Schweinhardt P, Seminowicz DA, Wood PB, Chizh BA, et al. "Accelerated Brain Gray Matter Loss in Fibromyalgia Patients: Premature Aging of the Brain?" *J Neurosci.* 2007; 27: 4004–4007.

[4] Walshe M. Mahasatipatthana Sutta. "The Long Discourses of the Buddha: A Translation of the Digha Nikaya." Boston: Wisdom Publications. 1987.

5 Anheyer D, Haller H, Barth J, Lauche R, Dobos G, Cramer H. "Mindfulness-Based Stress Reduction for Treating Low Back Pain: A Systematic Review and Meta-analysis." *Ann Intern Med.* 2017; 166(11): 799–807.

6 Cherkin DC, Sherman KJ, Balderson BH, et al. "Effect of Mindfulness-Based Stress Reduction vs Cognitive Behavioral Therapy or Usual Care on Back Pain and Functional Limitations in Adults With Chronic Low Back Pain: A Randomized Clinical Trial." *JAMA.* 2016; 315(12): 1240–1249.

7 Veehof MM, Trompetter HR, Bohlmeijer ET, Schreurs KM. "Acceptance- and Mindfulness-based Interventions for the Treatment of Chronic Pain: A Meta-Analytic Review." *Cogn Behav Ther.* 2016; 45(1): 5–31.

8 Cavanagh K, Strauss C, Forder L, Jones F. "Can Mindfulness and Acceptance be Learnt by Self-help?: A Systematic Review and Meta-analysis of Mindfulness and Acceptance-based Self-help Interventions." *Clin Psychol Rev.* 2014; 34(2): 118–129.

9 Ma X, Yue ZQ, Gong ZQ, et al. "The Effect of Diaphragmatic Breathing on Attention, Negative Affect and Stress in Healthy Adults." *Front Psychol.* 2017; 8: 874.

10 Holmes EA, Mathews A, Mackintosh B, Dalgleish T. "The Causal Effect of Mental Imagery on Emotion Assessed Using Picture-word Cues." *Emotion.* 2008; 8(3): 395.

11 Maples-Keller JL, Bunnell BE, Kim SJ, Rothbaum BO. "The Use of Virtual Reality Technology in the Treatment of Anxiety and Other Psychiatric Disorders." *Harv Rev Psychiatry.* 2017; 25(3): 103–113.

12 Zeidan F, Vago DR. "Mindfulness Meditation-based Pain Relief: A Mechanistic Account." *Ann N Y Acad Sci.* 2016; 1373(1): 114–127.

13 Pascoe MC, Thompson DR, Jenkins ZM, Ski CF. "Mindfulness Mediates the Physiological Markers of Stress: Systematic Review and Meta-analysis." *J Psychiatr Res.* 2017; 95: 156–178.

[14] Bakhshani NM, Amirani A, Amirifard H, Shahrakipoor M. "The Effectiveness of Mindfulness-Based Stress Reduction on Perceived Pain Intensity and Quality of Life in Patients With Chronic Headache." *Glob J Health Sci*. 2015; 8(4): 142–151.

[15] Herman PM, Anderson ML, Sherman KJ, Balderson BH, Turner JA, Cherkin DC. "Cost-effectiveness of Mindfulness-based Stress Reduction Versus Cognitive Behavioral Therapy or Usual Care Among Adults With Chronic Low Back Pain." *Spine (Phila Pa 1976)*. 2017; 42(20): 1511–1520.

[16] Anheyer D, Haller H, Barth J, Lauche R, Dobos G, Cramer H. "Mindfulness-Based Stress Reduction for Treating Low Back Pain: A Systematic Review and Meta-analysis." *Ann Intern Med*. 2017; 166(11): 799–807.

[17] Veehof MM, Trompetter HR, Bohlmeijer ET, Schreurs KM. "Acceptance- and Mindfulness-based Interventions for the Treatment of Chronic Pain: A Meta-analytic Review." *Cogn Behav Ther*. 2016; 45(1): 5–31.

CHAPTER 15: SLEEP SOUNDLY

[1] Dunietz GL, Swanson LM, Jansen EC, et al. "Key Insomnia Symptoms and Incident Pain in Older Adults: Direct and Mediated Pathways Through Depression and Anxiety." *Sleep*. 2018; 41(9).

[2] McCrae CS, Williams J, Roditi D, et al. "Cognitive Behavioral Treatments for Insomnia and Pain in Adults with Comorbid Chronic Insomnia and Fibromyalgia: Clinical Outcomes from the SPIN Randomized Controlled Trial." *Sleep*. 2019; 42(3).

[3] Yeung WF, Chung KF, Wong CY. "Relationship Between Insomnia and Headache in Community-based Middle-aged Hong Kong Chinese Women." *J Headache Pain*. 2010; 11(3): 187–195.

[4] Holbrook A, Crowther R, Lotter A, Endeshaw Y. "The Role of Benzodiazepines in the Treatment of Insomnia: Meta-analysis of

Benzodiazepine Use in the Treatment of Insomnia." J Am Geriatr Soc. 2001; 49(6): 824–826.

[5] Thakkar MM, Sharma R, Sahota P. "Alcohol Disrupts Sleep Homeostasis." *Alcohol*. 2015; 49(4): 299–310.

CHAPTER 16: TAME THE TOXINS

[1] Mostafalou S, Abdollahi M. "Pesticides and Human Chronic Diseases: Evidences, Mechanisms, and Perspectives." *Toxicol Appl Pharmacol*. 2013; 268(2): 157–177.

[2] Kim KH et al. "Exposure to Pesticides and the Associated Human Health Effects." *Sci Total Environment*. 2017; 575: 525–535.

CHAPTER 17: YOUR PAIN TREATMENT TOOLBOX

[1] Bednar DA, Orr FW, Simon GT. "Observations on the Pathomorphology of the Thoracolumbar Fascia in Chronic Mechanical Back Pain: A Microscopic Study." *Spine*. 1995; 20: 1161–1164

[2] Beardsley C, Skarabot J. "Effects of Self-myofascial Release: A Systematic Review. *J Bodyw Mov Ther*. 2015; 19(4): 747–58.

[3] Hotfiel T, Swoboda B, et al. "Acute Effects of Lateral Thigh Foam Rolling on Arterial Tissue Perfusion Determined by Spectral Doppler and Power Doppler Ultrasound." *J Strength Cond Res*. 2017; 31(4): 893–900.

[4] Qaseem A. et al. "Noninvasive Treatments for Acute, Subacute, and Chronic Low Back Pain: A Clinical Practice Guideline from the American College of Physicians." *Ann. Intern. Med*. 14 Feb, 2017.

[5] George D. et a. "Infrared for Chronic Low Back Pain: A Randomized, Controlled Trial." *Pain Research and Management*, Vol 11: 2006.

6 Salm DC, Belmonte LAO, Emer AA, Leonel LDS, de Brito RN, da Rocha CC, Martins TC, Dos Reis DC, Moro ARP, Mazzardo-Martins L, Kviecinski MR, Bobinski F, Salgado ASI, Cidral-Filho FJ, Martins DF. "Aquatic Exercise and Far Infrared (FIR) Modulates Pain and Blood Cytokines in Fibromyalgia Patients: A Double-Blind, Randomized, Placebo-Controlled Pilot Study." J Neuroimmunol. 2019 Dec 15; 337: 577077.

7 Baron EP. "Medicinal Properties of Cannabinoids, Terpenes, and Flavonoids in Cannabis, and Benefits in Migraine, Headache, and Pain: An Update on Current Evidence and Cannabis Science." Headache. 2018; 58(7): 1139–1186.

8 Boyaji, S., Merkow, J., Elman, R.N. et al. "The Role of Cannabidiol (CBD) in Chronic Pain Management: An Assessment of Current Evidence." Curr Pain Headache Rep 24, 4 (2020).

9 Überall MA. "A Review of Scientific Evidence for THC:CBD Oromucosal Spray (Nabiximols) in the Management of Chronic Pain." J Pain Res. 2020; 13: 399–410.

10 Capano A, Weaver R, Burkman E. "Evaluation of the Effects of CBD Hemp Extract on Opioid Use and Quality of Life Indicators in Chronic Pain Patients: A Prospective Cohort Study." Postgrad Med. 2020; 132(1): 56–61.

11 Piermarini C, Viswanath O. "CBD as the New Medicine in the Pain Provider's Armamentarium." Pain Ther. 2019; 8(1): 157–158.